THE BODYWORK BOOK

The enthusiastic response to Esme Newton-Dunn's lively keep-fit feature on the TVS afternoon magazine programme *Not For Women Only* has inspired Esme to write *The Bodywork Book*, in which she shows how to have fun while attaining a better, fitter body and an improved sense of well-being. The informative yet light-hearted style in which this book is written will prove a source of inspiration to both men and women, whatever their age, who are honest enough to admit that their bodies are not in the good condition they might be.

Chapters on every part of the body are included, together with exercises relating to each of those parts. *The Bodywork Book* also explains how to prevent and overcome common problems such as a weak back, flabby tummy muscles, rounded shoulders and fallen arches, and shows how to devise a personal exercise plan which will cater for your particular needs and capabilities.

In addition to her regular television appearances, Esme Newton-Dunn takes between 12 and 15 exercises classes each week at the Body Workshop Studio in West London. She also devised the exercises on *Cosmopolitan*'s 'Shape Tape 82'.

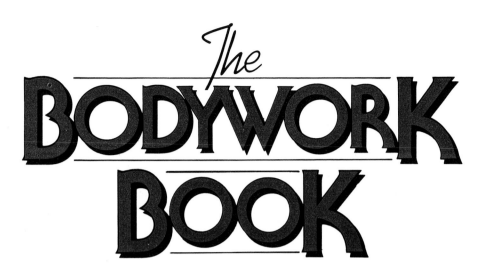

The BODYWORK BOOK

Esme Newton-Dunn

Illustrations by
NIGEL PAIGE

WILLOW BOOKS
Collins
St James's Place, London
1982

TO CLAYTON

Willow Books
William Collins Sons & Co Ltd
London · Glasgow · Sydney
Auckland · Toronto · Johannesburg

First published in Great Britain 1982
© TVS Ltd/Esme Newton-Dunn 1982

Jacket photography by Colin Thomas

Newton-Dunn, Esme
The bodywork book
1. Physical fitness
I. Title
613.7   RA776
ISBN 0 00 218007 3

Filmset in Baskerville by Ace Filmsetting Ltd, Frome
Printed in Great Britain by
William Collins Sons & Co Ltd Glasgow

Contents

My special thanks to John Miller of TVS for all his support and
for being instrumental in getting this book published; to all the
lovely people on *Not For Women Only* for their kindness; and to
Barbara Dale for all her help and time.

Whilst every care has been taken in the writing and compilation
of this book to ensure the exercises are as safe as possible, the
author and publisher cannot accept responsibility for any injury
sustained by the reader while doing the exercises. If you are in
any doubt as to your state of health, always consult a doctor
before embarking on an exercise programme.

Introduction

As a child I was plump, lazy and over indulged. My only interest in exercise was a craze for horses.

Things first began to go wrong when I bounced down iron stairs on my backside, which sent everyone into stitches but left me winded and with a smashed coccyx (tail bone). Although this was very painful no one seemed to be able to do much about it.

Then I started to develop breasts. They seemed to grow and grow but my height never reached 5ft 2in! So I rounded my shoulders in the hope that the breasts would disappear into a concave chest. As my shoulders hunched, my neck poked forwards and I must have greatly resembled a tortoise!

The final straw came when I had two bad riding falls and by the time I was fourteen I had slipped a disc in my neck. The muscles in my neck went into spasm, so I held my head permanently to one side. Eventually I was successfully treated but I felt that I should always have to be careful.

I came to loathe gym and games at school and tried to avoid them whenever possible. I gave up riding and tennis and became the ultimate unfit blob. I couldn't run ten yards without going puce in the face.

I managed to lose some weight after my first child – nerves I think – but the second baby left me fat and unfit. Clothes did not look good on me and I had little energy. I was certainly not happy with my body but resigned myself to it.

It was at that time that I met Barbara Dale, an ex-dancer who had studied many techniques before she discovered the Mensendeick method of gentle exercise, which many of the movements in this book are based on.

I became Barbara's first, worst and, finally, star pupil. Not that I enjoyed it at all at first; I was most reluctant to be dragged from my apathy, even once a week. It started to make sense when, after about a year, someone commented that I had changed shape – that did it! I was hooked and I had to admit that I also felt better.

I trained over the next five years, first working on my own body, then studying anatomy and physiology and how to exercise the body safely. I attended lectures on relaxation, nutrition, stress and anything related to keeping the body fit as a whole. I also took a course in massage, which I feel is a very healing treatment. I teach between two and five classes a day and this is where I continue to learn: it is through the people who come to my classes, each one with a body needing different attention, that I can better understand and help others to understand how to get back into shape.

Once you have grasped how to use your body, you will find that you develop a body awareness. This I think is vital. After all, it is how we sit, stand and move that shapes us, and good habits are far more effective than an hour's mindless workout a week, over and forgotten. It's no good going on a diet for a day and living on cream cakes for the rest of the week.

The final chapter of this book tells you how to put together some exercise programmes including warming up and down, so that once you've found your body awareness you can take it to whatever level you like.

1 Take a Good Look at Yourself

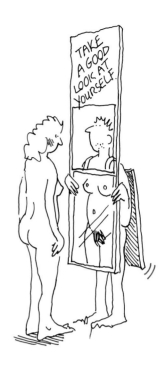

It amazes me how many people won't look at themselves in the mirror because they don't like what they see. Is it from guilt or a fear of being vain or, sadly, because they don't feel they live up to

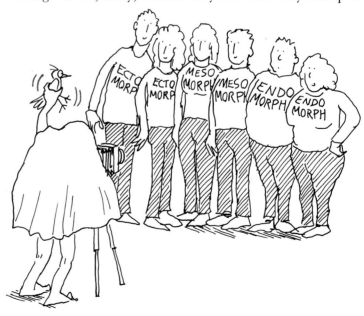

some mythical 'perfect shape' dreamed up by this year's fashion world?

Each of us fits loosely into one of three categories: *mesomorph* (that's me), *endomorph* and *ectomorph*. This means we have a basic body structure which we cannot change. If you are tall, and long to be short, forget it! Identify your basic body type and start accepting it.

1 *Mesomorph*
Excellent at fast and short-distance sports.

Sturdy, well muscled, yet agile. This type can go to seed, though, and end up flabby if the muscles are not used regularly.

2 *Ectomorph*
Good on stamina.

The willowy ones who make you sick because they can eat masses and stay thin – sometimes too thin.

3 *Endomorph*
Can spend hours in the swimming pool without feeling cold.

Cuddly bears put on weight easily and have to work hard to build muscle.

Remember that you are living in your body, and how you feel about it is going to affect your attitude to the world around you.

Book in hand, find the nearest FULL LENGTH mirror and get your clothes off! Now LOOK – back, front, sides, up and down.

Look at the way you are standing. Get a chair and sit on it the way you normally do, comfortably. Just keep observing; THIS IS YOU AS YOU ARE.

Is that tummy really all fat or do you stick it out when you are standing, slump when you are sitting?

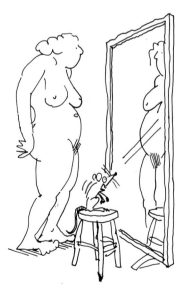

Some typical standing faults:

1 i Head pointing forwards, chin slightly up. (Squeezing the back of the neck.)

ii Shoulders up and rounded.

iii Sway back and tummy sticking out. (Squeezing the lower spine.)

iv Knees swayed back and turning in (knocked). (Not always together.)

v Feet turned slightly in and rolling onto inside edge.

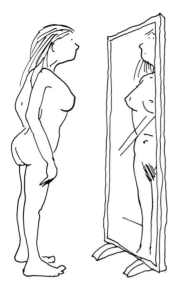

2 i Chin lifted (military bearing).

   ii Shoulders right back and chest
     pushed forwards.

  iii Back arched (*lordosis*).

  iv Knees locked back.

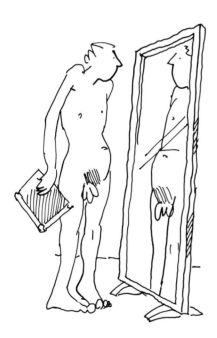

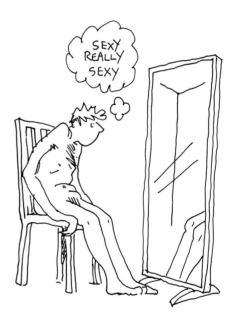

3 i Neck curved forwards
    (the droop).

  ii Rounded shoulders.

 iii Pelvis swayed forwards
    (*kyphosis*).

4 i Head tilted to one side.

  ii One shoulder up, one shoulder
    down, arms folded.

 iii Standing with one leg bent, the
    other straight so that one hip is
    up and one is down (*scoliosis* i.e.
    sideways curvature of the spine).
    (If left hip is up, right shoulder
    will be up to 'compensate'.)

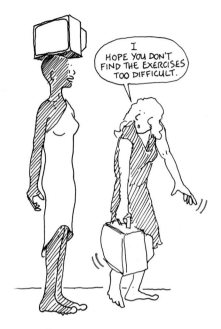

No one has a perfect body but you can improve and change your shape, sometimes dramatically, by using your body properly – like those wonderful African ladies who carry pots on their heads. Modern fast living does not allow us time to walk everywhere and all too often we are stuck behind the wheel of a car, or sitting for hours in a beautiful but horribly uncomfortable chair, or carrying heavy bags which nearly pull our arms out of their sockets, etc. If every movement we make exercises our body, think how many *bad* exercises we do every day! We have to counteract this first in order to get back to the basics.

You may also have a weight problem and this must be dealt with by both diet and exercise, and I do mean both. If you merely diet, especially if it is a crash diet, you are not going to maintain your weight loss for long and you enter into a constant up-and-down situation. It is extremely important to raise your metabolic rate through exercise. (Try running up the stairs instead of walking!) Once you have increased your metabolic rate, you will burn up the calories much more efficiently, thus being able to eat healthy amounts of food without always putting on weight. The bonus being that the more efficiently your body functions through exercise the less hungry you feel and the more energy you have. This book is about the basics of exercise though.

As far as diet goes this is the subject of another book I'm writing. Meanwhile think about this: our bodies are made up of cells which are constantly renewing themselves as the old cells die. The food we eat is building material for those cells. So before you reach for the junk and convenience foods just remember what you're building with.

Back to the mirror – you have taken a long look at yourself and got over the initial shock or admiration of what's on view. Next see in how many ways you correspond to the check list below – HONESTLY – and remember that what your body may *feel* is right may not correspond to what you *saw* in the mirror. Many people walk around completely lop-sided and yet think they are straight; when straightened up they feel lop-sided and can only be convinced by seeing themselves. Look for some of the compensations your body has to make in order to keep balanced. These can cause many problems such as curvature of the spine which, if not corrected, becomes more and more permanent.

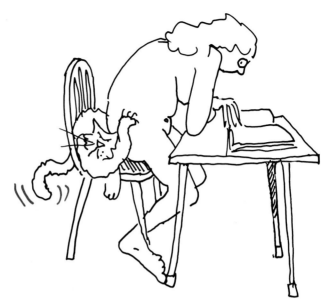

Some typical sitting faults:

1 (at a desk)

   i Hunched forwards, shoulders up, neck stuck out.

   ii Feet under chair and wrapped round leg of chair.

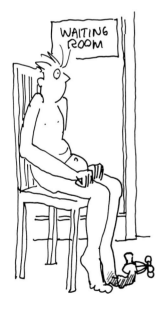

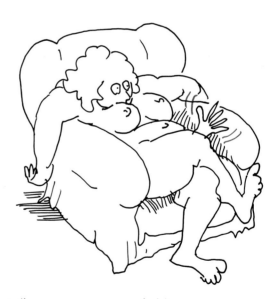

2 (in a waiting room)

   i Chair too high so legs dangling, toes resting on floor.

   ii Tensed up body, tight hands gripping bag or hat.

3 (in an enormous arm chair)

   i Completely slumped, legs all curled up.

   ii Everything squashed up!

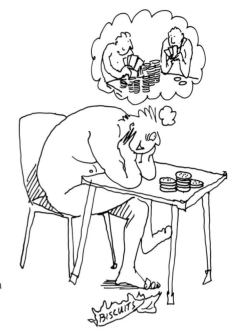

4 (at a table)

  i Leaning head on
    hands, propped up with
    elbows on table.

  ii Legs crossed.

HOW TO STAND PROPERLY

To stand properly, start with your feet – your foundation stones.

1 Your weight should fall evenly through your feet, with the central arch lifted, and a balance between your heels and the balls of your feet and your toes – like a tripod. Rock forwards onto the balls of your feet and back onto the heels to find the centre point of perfect balance.

2 Your knees should be soft, neither locked back nor bent.

3 Your bottom should be tucked under you – which will in turn pull in your tummy by centring your pelvis. You don't have to walk around with your buttocks clenched into a spasm and your tummy sucked in all day, but once you have strengthened them they will spring into place naturally. It is getting the correct positioning and having the awareness to *feel* when it's right that's important. (Repeated pelvic tilts will put this into practice – see pages 15 and 16.)

4 The centre of your body should be lifted between the hips and ribs, allowing plenty of space (for your newly pulled in tummy and all your digestive organs).

5 Your shoulders should fall down and into your back (not locked back) and line up with your hips and your ears. Try lifting your shoulders and moving them forwards and backwards and then dropping them into place.

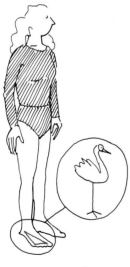

Standing properly –
'tripod' effect (*see* 1.)
and centred head (*see* 6.)

6 The back of your neck should be long with the chin at a right angle to your neck. Just nod your head gently forwards and backwards and then centre it.

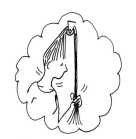

Standing properly – centred head (*see* 6.)

Now you should feel lifted and balanced – as if there is a string pulling up through the crown of your head. Your weight is evenly distributed through your muscles and you have lengthened and taken the pressure out of your spine. You should also be able to move in any direction from this position and not feel rigid like a robot.

Walk from your hips and allow your arms to swing freely. Try and walk through your feet; don't just plonk them on the ground or shuffle along. This is enough to depress anybody and put your body into a slump.

HOW TO SIT PROPERLY (Chart Ex. 1)

When sitting you should still feel lifted although now your weight-bearing joints are supported. Keep your legs parallel, and preferably hip width apart, with your feet slightly forwards to relax your calves. You should be able to feel two sitting bones in your bottom with your spine lengthening up from your pelvis. Try the following pelvic tilt, preferably sideways on to the mirror: put one hand on your tummy and one on your lower back; tilt or rock your hips back, pulling your tummy muscles in, and feel your back releasing. If you collapse or slump back you will feel your tummy bulge out. Next roll your hips forwards so you feel your back muscles pull in lifting your ribs at the same time so your tummy doesn't push forwards. In fact, your ribs should be lifted throughout this movement. This may sound quite simple but for many people it will seem impossible at first. Just keep trying because it will form the basis for so many movements. Once you feel you have mastered the backwards and forwards tilt, try doing them faster and then come back to the centre so there is a light tension or pull through the tummy and back muscles which will hold you lifted in the centre. Your shoulders should be relaxed with the back of the neck stretched upwards and the head poised confidently on top.

Back in your clothes again, take a look at your 'inner self'.

Do you often feel really tired and lethargic, do you suffer from the odd twinge? Perhaps your back frequently aches or your neck feels tight, but not enough to bother your doctor.

This book is about looking after yourself. Don't accept aches and pains as the norm and turn to pain killers as a way of life. If you had just bought a very expensive car, you would care for it and make sure it was serviced regularly – you can't just expect machinery to carry on without keeping its working parts tightened up and oiled. Our bodies are the most valuable and complex

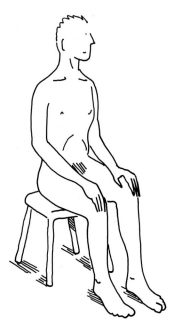

machine we will ever own, and yet because we take their miraculous workings for granted we only grumble and complain when they go wrong, without ever having thought about putting in a bit of time to maintain them and keep them in good working order.

When you reach for the aspirin bottle you are just 'covering up' the pain. There are times when this is necessary to allow the muscles to relax, but you are treating the *symptom* not the *cause*. Why have the muscles tensed up causing pain? I believe that even major illnesses can be avoided by using the body correctly and with understanding, maintaining a proper diet and controlling emotional stress.

Let's go through the body, area by area, working on the muscles and joints, finding strengths and weaknesses and getting everything back in place.

These gentle corrective exercises may be enough to keep you going on happily for ever, or you may find that with your new body awareness you would like to go on to some more energetic sports. But first things first. Each of the exercises in the book is numbered as a reference to the chart in Chapter 9, which puts together an hour's exercise routine.

Sitting properly – legs parallel and hip width apart, feet forwards, calves relaxed

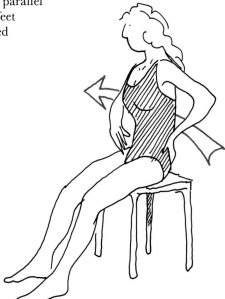

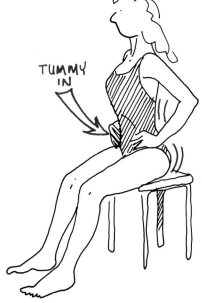

Pelvic tilt – the backwards tilt – the pelvis tilting backwards – tummy pulling in

The forwards tilt – back pulling in, ribs lifted

16

2 The Amazing Balancing Act

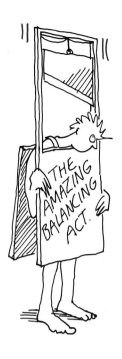

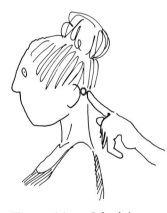

The position of the joint on which your head nods

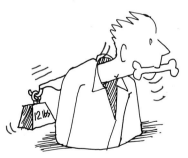

The 'nodding dog' look

Your head weighs 10–12 lb and balances on top of the first seven vertebrae of your spine. Through these vertebrae pass all the nerves that supply your body, from your heart to your big toe. Also passing through your neck is the vital blood supply to and from your brain.

The joint on which your head nods backwards and forwards is underneath the bulge at the base of the skull (occipital bones). If you put your finger into the hollow under your skull and move your head gently backwards and forwards you should be able to feel this. It is also the point from which you should lengthen your neck, not by lifting your chin.

If your neck pokes forward it has the appearance of bending from the base of the neck – rather like one of those nodding dogs. This not only looks rather unattractive, but try to imagine the strain it is putting on the muscles that are trying to support your neck.

Worse still, when your neck starts to poke forwards it drags the shoulders up after it so that they round up and forwards and this sets up a whole pattern of compensation for the rest of your spine.

Think for a moment about gravity – what goes up must come down. Well, gravity is what keeps our feet firmly planted on the ground, but it is also pulling at the rest of us all the time. If you stand a pencil on its end, gravity will pass straight through the centre of it and it will balance. If you try to stand it at an angle, it will be pulled down by gravity. We are not rigid pencils but bendy bodies, so when we push a part of ourselves off centre, instead of toppling over we bend somewhere else to compensate. I have illustrated some of the compensatory curves in Chapter 1. Now, starting at the top, I hope to help you understand how these curves happen and to give you some practical ways of getting them back into balance again. If you can get the spine right from the top vertebra, by lengthening the neck then lifting the chest and dropping the shoulders, the rest will follow.

When you lift your head try to imagine that there is a string pulling up through the crown of your head and that it is pulling up and up. This is not lifting your chin up, which only tilts your head back shortening and tightening the muscles at the back of your neck. Short people have to spend quite a lot of time lifting their chins up and some cinemas have their screens raised so that you have to look upwards. If you are in a situation where you have had your head held back for some time, compensate by allowing it to 'stretch' forwards, as described below. After lengthening your neck you should no longer feel stiff and rigid! The neck should be long, strong and mobile.

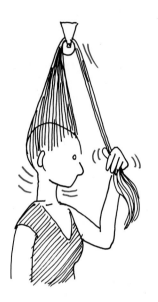

Imagine a string pulling up and up as you lift your head

RELAXING AND STRENGTHENING THE NECK
(Chart Ex. 5)

The first thing is to test how much tension there actually is up the back of your neck. This is going to change throughout the day,

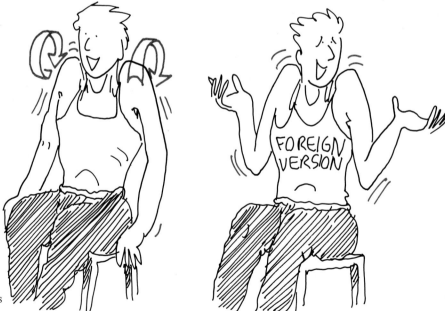

Shoulder circles

so you have to use your body 'awareness' to tell you when things begin to tighten up. Then you can release the tension before it builds up into something more serious such as pain, stiffness and headache.

This is best done sitting on a firm chair or stool, so before we start it is important that you sit correctly (see Chapter 1, correct sitting). First, to make sure your shoulders are dropping down away from ears, do this shoulder movement: Lift your shoulders up towards your ears and then pull them back – just your shoulders, don't arch your back as well. Now lower them (without collapsing in the middle), keeping your neck long, and then release them. Try this several times, then put these movements together into a shoulder circle. (See page 27 Chart Ex. 2) If you hear grinding and cracking, there is too much tension around the joints and they need loosening up. (See Chapter 3 on shoulders.)

FIRST NECK POSITION (Chart Ex. 3)

Leave your shoulders down, tuck in your chin and then let your head gently tilt forwards. This is the *first neck position*. You may feel a pull up the back of your neck straight away. If it is not too strong, go on to the second stage:

Loosely clasp your hands together and rest them on the knob at the back of your head (with your head still in the first neck position) letting your arms relax so that your elbows are hanging on either side of your face. The more you relax your arms the heavier they become. Each arm weighs about 10 lb. Add this to the weight

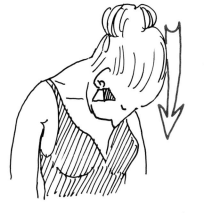

Relaxing the neck – first neck position

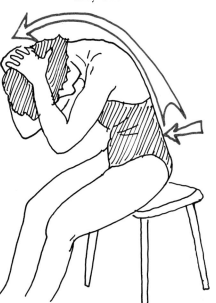

Relaxing the neck – curling the body around an imaginary ball to release tension down spine

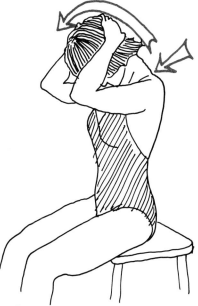

Relaxing the neck – 'releasing tension out' with the added weight of the arms

of your head and you will understand why this gives you such a good stretch. If you are a very tense person you may find it hard to relax. You will find your elbows are lifted and you will be tempted to try tugging down on the head to pull that tension out. DON'T EVER, EVER JERK OR TUG AT THE HEAD IN THIS WAY. This is a passive stretch, and the muscles must be allowed to RELAX in order to stretch out and release that tension. What muscle is ever going to relax if you are forcing and tugging at it? Apart from the damage you could do, remember that when a muscle is tense it goes hard and knotted, it is in spasm. Hard mean brittle, soft means pliable – this applies to all the muscles of your body.

Now I hope you've got the message about just hanging there with your head relaxed forwards and your arms adding extra weight to increase the stretch. Try to soften your face too. Make sure you are not clenching your teeth and that your jaw is relaxed, soften your tongue, close your eyes. Take a deep breath in and let it out slowly – like a sigh of relief, to help you release and let go.

If the stretch becomes too much, bring your head up and then try again; or take away the weight of your arms and go back to the first position. If, however, you feel little or no pull, you can go into the third stage which takes the stretch down from the back of the neck into the muscles that run on either side of the spine (*spinus rectae*). In some people tension occurs, not in the neck, but lower down, often between the shoulder blades. When you reach this tension point, you will feel a 'block' in that spot. 'Hang' at this level until you begin to feel a release – but don't overdo the hanging. Start off for just a minute or two and build up.

For the third stage tilt your hips back and pull in your tummy muscles as you did in the pelvic tilting for correct sitting. Now imagine there is a large beach ball resting on your lap and curl your body up and over it. You may not be able to go very far before you reach your block. The further forwards you go the further down the spine you will feel the stretch. Uncurl slowly and lower your arms.

Always do the first 'test' position before you go into any further stages and you can use the first neck position in almost any situation during the day if you become aware of tension beginning to build up, i.e. your shoulders are beginning to rise up to your ears and you feel a tightness coming into your neck – it doesn't even have to look as if you are doing an 'exercise'! Try to keep your neck long and your shoulders down all the time.

When your neck feels tender and aches it is always beneficial to gently massage it. Start with the pads of muscles at the base of the neck and draw the flesh forwards over the top of your shoulders. You can also work over these muscles with a circular movement of the fingers. They are the root of the neck (*trapezius*) muscles. Now tilt your head into the first neck position (chin tucked in) and then starting at the knob at the base of your neck (seventh cervical vertebra) run your fingers up on either side of

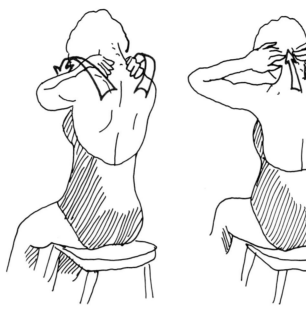

Relaxing the neck – working base of
neck muscles with circular finger
movements

Relaxing the neck – upwards
massage in first neck position

the spine pushing gently and firmly upwards until you reach the
bulge of the skull (occipital bones). Let your fingers slide lightly
down the sides of your neck so that you don't lose contact and
then push upwards again. (Any lumps and bumps are knots of
tension, so pause to work on them to knead away the knots.) This
helps to push the blood upwards to the brain (against gravity).
When you feel a headache coming on the emphasis of the massage
should be reversed so that the pressure is downwards. This is because the muscles of the neck, as they tighten over squeeze the
blood vessels, trapping blood in the head. This causes pressure
which can be released by drawing the blood downwards and away
from the head. When your headache gets really bad your best bet
is a pain killer which will allow the muscles to relax as the pain
lessens. This only treats the symptom, not the cause, so try to avoid
neck-tension which causes headaches! For persistent headaches
consult your doctor.

Keep your scalp loose too by massaging it – when washing your
hair is a good time. Instead of just scrubbing at the hair try to
move the scalp slowly over your skull.

It's all very well having these amazingly pliable muscles, but
where does the strength to hold your head up come from? I've
talked a lot about tension as a bad thing, but in fact without a
certain amount of tension in our muscles we would all be floppy
blobs and with no tension in the back of our necks our heads would
just loll on our chests. Tension only becomes a problem when we

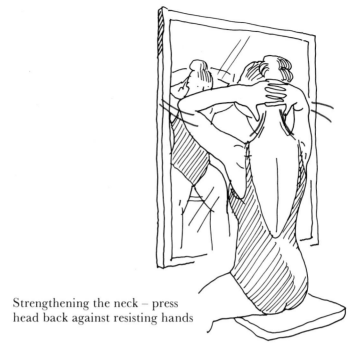

Strengthening the neck – press
head back against resisting hands

get too much of it and we can't let go of it, so it builds up and
becomes spasm! This is negative tension.

Muscles work in pairs to move joints, so every time one set of
muscles pulls (tenses) the opposite set of muscles must release
(relax) in order to allow movement. Our bodies are constantly
shifting and adjusting states of pulls and releases. Some muscles
are almost permanent 'pullers', and these are the ones we have to
guard against holding too much of that pull (tension). The back
of the neck is a very good case in point. It has to keep your heavy
head lifted and moving, against the pull of gravity, all day. What
we must be careful of here is not to mix weakness with tension.
Normally and with everything working properly, controlled
tension should correspond with strength (this is positive tension)
but if your neck is weak and it can't hold your head upright then
it will poke forwards putting even more stress into those muscles
which can only hold the head by going into spasm (negative
tension). *See* illustration 'Nodding Dog' page 17.

NECK STRENGTHENER (Chart Ex. 5)

This is how to keep the muscles at the back of your neck strong
enough to hold it upright with the minimum of positive tension:

Loosely clasp your hands on the knob at the back of your head
and allow your elbows to fall outwards. Now tuck in your chin
so the back of your neck is very straight. Don't allow your head to
poke forwards or downwards. Look straight ahead and press your
head back whilst resisting with your hands. The movement is very
small. You can feel the top part of the muscles working by resting
your thumbs down on your neck. Only hold this 'squeeze' for a

few seconds and then release. Repeat this movement several times. You may be horrified to see double or even multiple chins appearing when you tuck in your chin and these get even worse as you press back. Don't worry! Double chins come from weakness at the back of the neck which allows everything to fall forwards (pulled by gravity again). If the muscles at the back of the neck are strong enough they will 'pull back' everything from the front. Here again, you must look at your basic jaw structure. Maybe your jaw is more prone to double chins than someone else's, in which case I can't promise that you won't get a double chin in your old age – but it won't be such a bad one. If you've got them

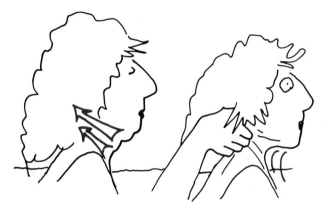

Strengthening the neck muscles will help get rid of double chins

already, they could improve! And when the back of your neck is strong you will be able to keep it long, which makes it look better anyway.

If the back of your neck was exceptionally tight in the first position, get rid of some of this tightness before you try the strengthening exercise. After all you don't want to seize up! Everything should be balanced between strength and suppleness.

You will notice that the chin is tucked in for all the neck exercises – for the amount of time you tuck your chin in you will not get any extra chins, as explained, but it will keep your neck long and straight to protect your vertebrae while you exercise your neck muscles. There should, however, be a slight natural curve in the back of the neck as in the lower back, so it is just as bad to keep your chin pulled in all the time as it is to let your head droop forwards. Pulling in your chin all day to lengthen the back of your neck would certainly produce double chins and is not the right position. (The chin should be held at a right angle to your neck.)

The more you use your muscles (correctly!) the more easily they should spring back into place, thus requiring very little effort to hold everything together. It's all about getting into the right habits.

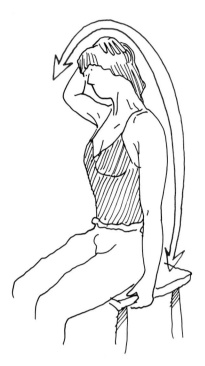

Side neck release

SIDE RELEASE (Chart Ex. 4)

These are two other releases for the neck:

Start by tucking in your chin, then tilt your head over to the side starting to the right (once you know what you are doing, which side you start on is not important) and anchor your left shoulder down by holding on to the leg of the chair directly below your shoulder. (You may have to sit slightly forward to achieve this.) Rest your right hand on your head so that the fingers are just above your left ear. Relax your arm so that it adds weight to the head and you feel a stretch up the left side of your neck. Make sure there is a space between your right ear and shoulder and that you are not hunching up the shoulder. Your left arm is now pulling down your left shoulder, which is one end of the muscle, and your right arm is adding weight to the direction of the head, thus drawing out the other end of the muscle (mainly sterno mastoid). As your right arm is a weight it must line up with the muscle which is drawing out, so make sure the elbow stays out to the side. You should feel a long (strong, if the muscle is tight) stretch from the shoulder to behind the ear. The less you feel the better. To increase the stretch keep pulling down with the left hand without tilting your body and tuck your chin in more. If you feel the stretch concentrated in only one spot, this is a 'block'. Stretch in this direction for a minute or two and then repeat on the other side. (Right arm down, tilt head to the left, add weight of left arm, pull in chin).

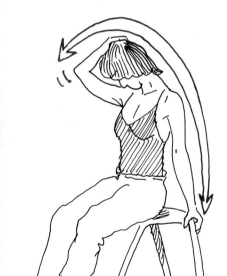

Diagonal neck release

DIAGONAL NECK RELEASE (Chart Ex. 6)

Put your left hand down and back, and hold on to the back leg of the chair with the palm of your hand rotated forwards so that your shoulder stays down and back and doesn't roll up and forwards. Turn your head to the right halfway towards your right shoulder. Tuck in your chin and tilt your head forwards until you feel a stretch up from your left shoulder narrowing up into your neck. If this isn't too strong, add your right arm to your head, letting your elbow flop by the side of your face, for weight. To increase the stretch take the head further forwards and pull down more with your left arm on the chair. Come up slowly and repeat on the other side. Right arm down and back, turn head diagonally to the left and tilt forwards then add left arm.

If you feel persistent tightness in the same spot, you must look at the way you are holding your head or at what you are doing during the day. Some of the strains we put on ourselves cannot be helped, so the only way to deal with them is to compensate by doing a stretch to draw out the tight spot. But perhaps some of the things you do are not really necessary – such as tucking your telephone under one ear and holding it in place by lifting your shoulder (if you have to do it, at least try to change sides every now and again), or always copy-typing from the same side (prop the paper straight in front of you or, again, change sides). Keep looking at the little things you do habitually, without thinking –

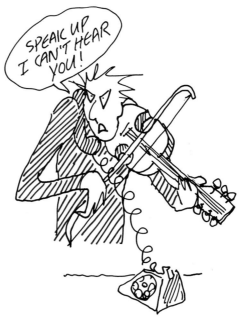

because they have become second nature to you, you frequently don't notice the slow build up of tension before it becomes pain.

Try to avoid circular head movements. Rolling the weight of your head, pulled down by gravity, and made worse if the muscles are tight squashes the vertebrae closer together. HEAD CIRCLES CAN GRIND YOUR VERTEBRAE. Avoid all violent movements of the head. If you want to test mobility, bring your head gently forwards and then backwards (keeping the back of the neck lengthened and not allowing the head to 'flop' back), tilt the head from side to side and then rotate (turn) it from side to side. This is the amazing range of movement we have in our neck, in spite of the immense weight it is having to bear.

I start every one of my classes with these exercises, however hard I expect people to work afterwards. The neck is a weak spot and it is no good doing stronger exercises when the back of your neck is knotted up. You will inevitably find that the strain starts to creep into your neck and it is only through awareness that you can correct this.

3 Shouldering Your Problems

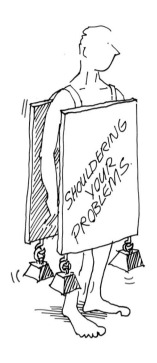

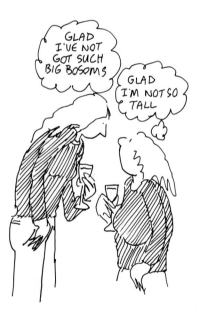

Psychological problems can become physical problems

In this chapter it is important to look at some of the causes of 'bad' shoulders. I have already mentioned why I developed round shoulders. Tall people often stoop in order to make themselves look shorter (they usually end up drawing more attention to themselves).

These are psychological reasons for rounding shoulders, but there is also an important physiological one. Almost every arm movement we make is forwards, and arms are closely involved with shoulders. In fact the shoulder joint has the widest range of movement – think of how many ways you can lift and turn your arms. The shoulder blades themselves 'float' in muscle in order to allow this freedom of movement, so if the muscles become stretched from always pulling forwards naturally the shoulder blades will open out. Anything you leave long enough will eventually become worse and stay so. This is why people develop stoops and dowager's humps! This type of problem can be dealt with by strengthening the muscles that support the shoulder blades, in order to pull them back into place. This is done by 'shoulder squeezes', which are important for everyone because of the amount of forward movements we make – driving, washing up, writing and many other everyday activities. Some people's work involves an acceleration of this problem, which may also include lifting the shoulders. Think of dentists, hairdressers, secretaries, Mums feeding their babies – all hunched up over their work (have a look at some well known tennis players too!).

So where should the shoulders be? They should fall below the ears so that the shoulder blades are flat into the back and the shoulders slope downwards. Have a look at your collar bones in the mirror. If they are more or less straight across, then your shoulders are down and back as they should be. If they are up at an angle with hollows, then your shoulders are where they *shouldn't* be.

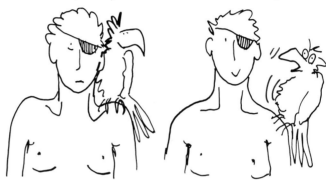

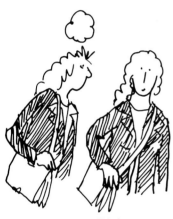

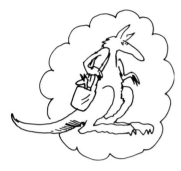

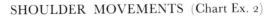
Shouldering your problems – wrong way, right way

Wrong way   Right way

Before I go any further, I would like to mention shoulder bags. Not just the kind women carry, but any bag carried on the shoulders from the photographer's to long-handled shopping baskets (they don't even have to be specially heavy). If your shoulders are supposed to slope downwards, anything you hang on them is not going to stay there long; it is going to slide off. So what do you do in order to keep it there? Of course, you have to lift your shoulder! If it's something very, very heavy you are probably going to change shoulders every now and again in order to take some of the pressure off; but if it's a reasonably light bag which you always carry, you'll probably find you get into the habit of always wearing it on the same side. And very subtly your shoulder will lift to keep it there, then they become fixed there so that those muscles will retain that negative tension. People often complain that they have pain on one side of their neck and shoulder, and the shoulder bag is one of the major causes! So why not get rid of it and start again, or if you can't afford to change your bag for another, at least try and adapt it to a hand or clutch bag. Alternatively, try wearing it across you as this takes the weight off your shoulder, or if you *have* to carry it at least make sure you change shoulders frequently!

SHOULDER MOVEMENTS (Chart Ex. 2)

Start by raising your shoulders and then letting them drop down. Just carry on lifting and dropping, and then rest. Now lift again and then move them backwards and forwards. Keep your tummy in while you do this as you only want to move your shoulders, not your whole body! Drop them down again and then combine these movements. Bring your shoulders forward, lift them up, take them back and then down. Repeat this a few times as separate movements and then quicken them up and you'll find you are circling your shoulders backwards as you did before you took your head forwards in Chart Ex. 5. Try to make big circles, going through each point every time, and then relax the shoulders down again. I am emphasising the backwards movement to counteract the forwards movements we already do, but there is nothing wrong with a few forward circles if you feel the need. Was there any clicking or crunching going on as you circled your shoulders? This is caused by tension and I will be dealing with your shoulders under stress later in this chapter. Meanwhile just keep moving those shoulders up and down, backwards and forwards, and circling to try and ease up the muscles.

Another quick deviation here. If you have to carry heavy things – suitcases, parcels, briefcases, shopping – do you ever feel as if your shoulder has been pulled out of its socket? Or perhaps feel slight numbness or tingling in the fingers? (If numbness or tingling in the arm or hand persist you must check with your doctor.) Carrying very heavy weights can pull on the nerve supply to the arm (*brachial plexus*). This stretch on the nerve is the cause of the pain. To alleviate it just do the opposite to pulling down and take the pressure off by lifting your shoulders and folding your arms and either resting them on your chest or a table.

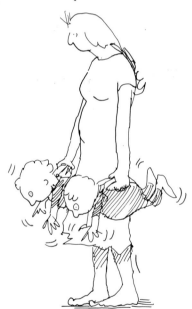

Carrying heavy weights can cause pain

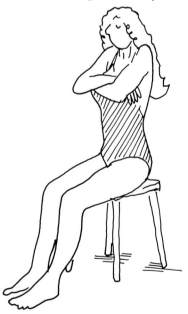

Shoulder release – alleviating painfully stretched nerves (by lifting shoulders and supporting folded arms)

If there was not too much scrunching going on in your shoulders, you could try doing some arm swings standing up. You can of course do all the shoulder exercises standing, but I prefer to do them sitting as the body is supported and you can concentrate more on the relevant part. Seated arm swings are a bit awkward, so when you stand do make sure your bottom is tucked well underneath you and that your back does not arch everytime your arm goes back. Starting with one arm at a time, just swing it back and go through a full circle with your finger tips making sure that you brush past the side of your head each time. Then both together – expect this to be much stronger and your arms soon to feel warm and tired. These circles are all designed to loosen up around the joint, and they are included in the warm-ups in Chapter 7 page 114. The next exercises set to work on specific muscle groups, these are the shoulder squeezes.

SHOULDER SQUEEZE (Chart Ex. 9)

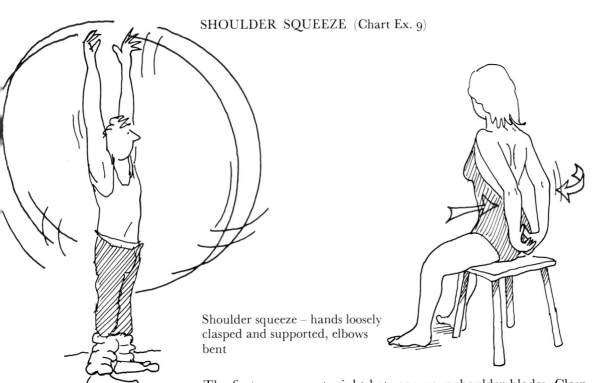

Shoulder squeeze – hands loosely clasped and supported, elbows bent

Shoulder release – arm-swings standing up

The first squeeze gets right between your shoulder blades. Clasp your hands loosely – look at the illustration – and rest them on your bottom or lower back, keeping your elbows bent. It is important to keep your elbows bent so that you can use your upper arm to squeeze back (with straight arms you can only go back the width of your body). Press the elbows back towards each other making sure that your hands stay where they are and that your shoulders pull together and don't shoot up! Very occasionally you find someone whose shoulder joints are loose enough to allow their elbows to come together. Don't worry about this (although there is a later exercise – the chicken – where you will have to be careful).

This exercise should be done as a strong squeeze, then a release, and then repeated. When you are trying to strengthen muscles it is not advisable to hold a contraction for too long. If a muscle is held tightly contracted in one position for too long, that tension begins to build up in a negative way. Positive tension is when the muscle springs back into place. It is firm but elastic. Negative tension is the kind I mentioned earlier, the kind we associate with pain, tightness, spasm. So don't overdo your shoulder squeeze and think that, if you hold it for half an hour, your shoulders will stay back. They won't and you'll end up with a sore back!

It takes a long time for your body to slip out of alignment and also time to put it back. You started pulling your shoulders forward from the day you were put behind a school desk! Little and often is the most effective way to work; I have written this book in such a way that you can take a bit out and put it into your everyday life, rather than feel that if you miss doing your sequence of exercises you might as well leave the whole lot until tomorrow and tomorrow!

You will normally want to pull back after a long bout of forwards movements; so here's an exercise to get you back into balance again.

The next squeeze is much stronger and you must be careful not to let it put any negative tension back into your neck. If you do feel tension building up, always let your head go forwards to keep the muscles stretched – don't lift your shoulders and take your head back, thereby tightening the muscles still further. With luck you won't feel too much in your neck, so you will be able to keep your head straight upright.

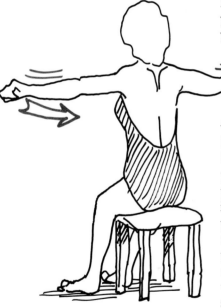
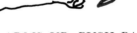

ARMS UP, PUSH BACK (Chart Ex. 7)

Raise your arms to shoulder level, keeping your shoulders down. Make a loose fist with your hands (this adds weight to the end of your arms), squeeze your shoulder blades together (don't arch your back, so keep your pelvis centred!), and push your arms back in small progressive movements. At first you won't be able to hold your arms up for long and you will feel it mainly in your upper arm. So when your arms get tired just bring them down and circle your shoulders back to release them. As you begin to use your upper back more, you will find that you are able to distribute the weight of the arm through these muscles, making the whole area stronger.

Arms up, push back

Once you feel you are getting on well with this first movement, go on to the next stage. Don't forget to let your head tilt forwards if you feel tension coming into your neck; leave it out if your neck is a real problem – get rid of the negative tension in your neck first!

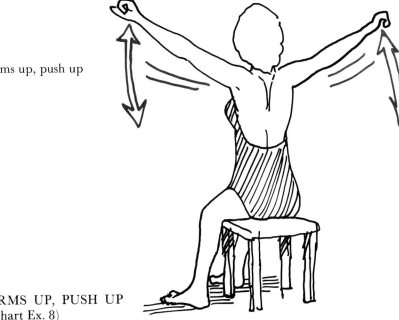

Arms up, push up

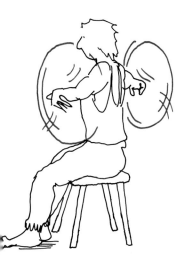

Arms up – combining movements 1. and 2. to make small backwards circles

ARMS UP, PUSH UP
(Chart Ex. 8)

Lift the arms again and squeeze your blades together as you did before. This time, keeping your blades together and your shoulders down, lift your arms in small further movements. This is harder, as you are pulling down your shoulders as you push up your arms! Take a rest and circle your shoulders to release. If you combine these two movements, you get small backwards circles emphasising the up and back movements.

Don't overdo these exercises, especially at first, but don't give up too quickly either. Try to build up until you can keep going long enough to feel the muscles glow.

You have now worked the centre and top of the shoulders. This next exercise (I call it 'the chicken') works on the muscles that stretch diagonally down across the back from behind the arms to the waist. The bulk of these muscles (*latissimus dorsi*) form a girdle from below the shoulder blades to waist level; they are vital for good posture and you will come across them again later. For the moment we are only concerned with a small part of them, a sort of tail end that goes up into the back of your arm. This part of the muscle isn't used much (which is why you have to do such a peculiar exercise to get at it), so it can get weak and flabby. It is particularly noticeable in older women wearing sleeveless dresses – these are the muscles that go to flab.

THE 'CHICKEN' (Chart Ex. 10)

To prevent or contain the deterioration of these muscles, rest your hands on your ribs with your elbows bent. Pull your shoulders down and then take your elbows back with a quick firm movement (now you know why I call it 'the chicken'). Just keep flapping your wings, but with deliberation not sloppily! You can do some slower movements, then speed them up a bit. Feel your shoulders pull together and squeeze where the arm joins the back.

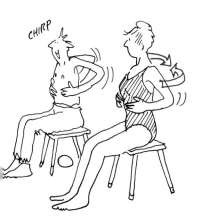

Doing the 'chicken', hands on ribs, elbows bent

31

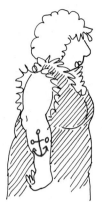

THE BACK OF THE ARM TIGHTENER (Chart Ex. 11)

The other area which can get loose and flabby is the muscle under the arm. Again, you find this particularly in women as men's arms tend to be stronger. With your arms hanging down by your sides make your hands into loose fists, then turn your arms inwards until the back of your hand is facing forwards and then in a bit more. Keep your shoulders down and bending from the elbows throw your arms straight back, keeping your upper arm close in to your side, and repeat several times. What should happen is that, as your arm straightens back, the back of the arm tightens up. Your arms should not be able to fly too far back as the shoulders are holding down to block this.

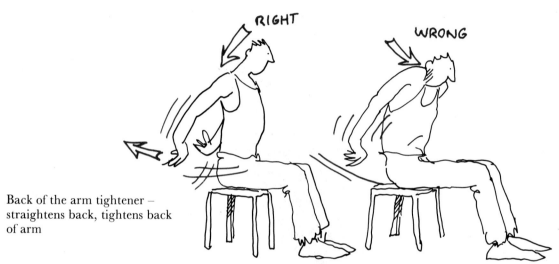

Back of the arm tightener –
straightens back, tightens back
of arm

What happens, if your shoulders pop up and forwards as your arms go back, is a feeble and useless movement! The backs of our arms weaken because we spend more time bending them forwards. As joints are moved by pairs of muscles, one set shortening the other stretching in order to allow movement, the backs of the arms spend a lot of time being stretched, in the same way as the shoulders are always reaching forwards.

To increase the strength of this exercise keep the arms straight and slightly back and then push further back in quick movements concentrating the tightening effect.

ARM ROTATION (Chart Ex. 12)

To release your arms and to rotate the arm in the shoulder socket stretch your arms out to the sides of your body, about a quarter of the way up. Turn your hand, palm upwards, stretching out through your fingers at the same time. Try to bring your little finger up to the top and round. You will feel your shoulders pulling down into your back as you do this movement. Now reverse it,

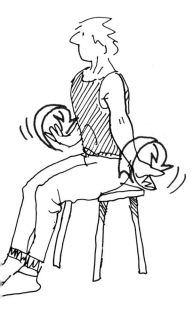

Arm rotation – shoulders must be kept down and back

rotating the arm forwards and trying to bring your thumb uppermost. You will feel your shoulders wanting to follow your arms round – hold them down and back! Stretch through your fingers all the time you are turning your arms to keep the muscles tight and strong. Rotate them backwards and forwards several times, bending them fully between each rotation. It is when you lose this rotation and the ability to take your arm back that you find you can no longer get your arm back into the sleeve of your coat. Keep all joints mobile!

Now you've got your shoulders pulling back, do make sure you don't get carried away and walk around with your chest stuck forwards and back arched like a sergeant major! It's all a matter of balance and once you have strengthened the muscles they should spring back into place normally, with only a few reminders from you to keep them there.

The position you find your shoulders in is only a symptom. We have looked at some of these, both psychological and physiological, now I want to look at your shoulders under stress. Stress is such a huge subject that I can only touch on it here, but I have chosen to put it in now as the shoulders are such a good barometer of stress.

Stress, like tension, is not the evil we have come to accept. If there was not stress in our lives where would be our impetus, our energy, our ambition? Stress releases adrenaline. Some people thrive on it, taking each new challenge in their stride. Other people have a very low stress tolerance and each new problem sends them into a state. Stress changes the chemical balance of the body and puts it into an emergency state. Everyone knows what panic feels like, but how does it manifest itself physically? Have you ever seen a happy person hunched up in a corner – arms folded, clenched fists, feet wrapped around the leg of the chair and shoulders up round their ears?

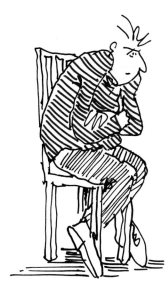

Unhappiness is a hunched, tight, in-turned body

Happiness is loose, free and open, so what happens when we take on more stress than we can cope with? Primitive man used flight or fight. The kind of pressures that our ancestors had to face were fairly basic; if they were under attack, they either ran like hell or turned round and fought it out. This meant that the chemical effects of stress and all the waste products which accumulate with an energy surge were worked off physically. Now, when you are stuck in a traffic jam and are late for a meeting, you don't get out and beat up the driver of the car in front. When you have a row on the telephone, you don't rip it out of its socket and kick it round the room. If someone puts you down and is really mean and rotten to you, do you run away? No, you just stay and store it all up in yourself. With all this pent up energy inside you, is it surprising that your shoulders shoot up? Sometimes a good verbal exchange and a bit of arm waving will do the trick; sometimes we need to go away somewhere quiet to try and relax, slow down the breathing and the heart rate, rationalise. Or we turn to a physical way of working things off: jogging, tennis, squash, something all absorbing and energy consuming, so that we're too tired to care about our problem anymore!

First, isolate the cause of your stress. You'll know it's there by the state of your body. You cannot separate body and mind, so if your neck is tight and your shoulders are round your ears there's something wrong. It may be an isolated problem or it may be something that's there all the time. Traffic noise, someone getting at you subtly all the time, the neighbours' dogs! Then evaluate yourself and how you are best physically suited to dealing with the problem. If you are fat and very unfit, don't choose jogging to start with. If you spend your life behind a desk and haven't played squash for ten years, don't think that the odd game is going to do the trick – it could do you more harm than good; even kill you, without proper preparation. You may have built up so much stress in your body that you are unable to sit down for five minutes or sleep at night – you need to learn to relax before you should even think of doing anything physical that will only compound your tension.

Yet ultimately we should all be able to work off our stress physically (back to the 'fight or flight') because this is how to get rid of the waste products I mentioned: the fatty acids which, if they are not burned up, remain in the blood stream, silting up arteries and depositing fat around the vital organs.

Start by *preparing* and *understanding* your body with this book. You should find that as you loosen your joints it will help you to relax them too. Join a fitness centre or a dance class. Read a book on jogging or running so that you can do it properly. Skip, swim, or bicycle; anything to get you moving again. Whatever you do choose, make it something that you enjoy and which stretches your capabilities. You have a duty to look after the body you were given, so put it at the top of your priority list, not as something that can be left until next week. Fitness affects you mentally and physically and how you feel affects everything from your relationships to your ability to cope. Get the most out of life, so that you can give your best.

4 Back to the Bottom

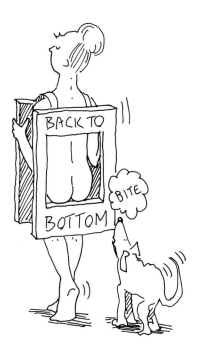

Gluteus maximus, *medius* and *minimus*. These are the muscles which make up the most fleshy part of our body, our bottom. They come in all shapes and sizes from the almost non-existent to the vast and spreading mass, but what are they doing there in the first place?

No, they are not just sexy little things to wiggle as you walk, although that may well be a part of their design! They are there to help support the back and the weight of the pelvis. In some primitive tribes they also acted as a food store, but here we are just dealing with getting them shaped up and back in their place.

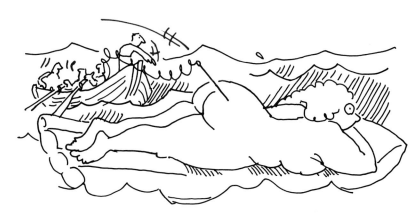

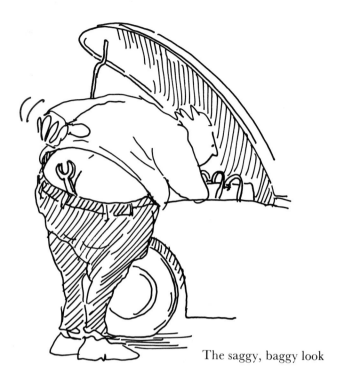

The saggy, baggy look

When you took a look at yourself in the mirror, how was the lower half of your body looking? Did your back curve inwards? Did your bottom spread round to your hips? Did it droop at the back? Was it all flabby and saggy and sad?

Don't stop reading this chapter if the answer to all these questions is no! If you've got a lovely, round, tight little bottom and you aim to keep it that way, this applies to you too!

The most important thing I have said so far is that your bottom is there to help support your lower back and pelvis. When you squeeze your buttocks together, something magical happens: your pelvis centres and your tummy muscles pull in. THIS IS THE AMAZING PELVIC TILT! Most tilting exercises will in fact come in the next chapter because the pelvic is tipped back by pulling in the tummy. What squeezing your buttocks has done is put your pelvis back in place under you instead of letting it tilt forwards. Look at the illustrations to see what I mean.

You cannot separate the action of the buttocks from that of the tummy muscles on the tilt of the pelvis; weak buttock and back muscles cause lower back problems, as do weak tummy muscles too. This area must pull as a whole to work effectively. The lower back curve, like the neck curve, is vital but vulnerable. Over-exaggerate that curve or lose it altogether (which is less common) and you are laid open to problems. Many backs have become so fixed and rigid that, clench as you may on your buttocks, there

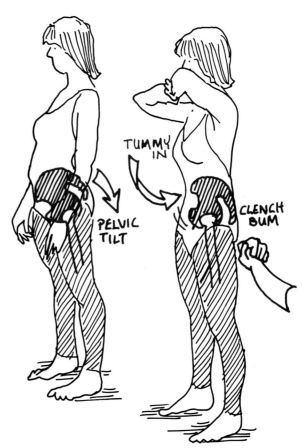

The amazing pelvic tilt – centreing the pelvis

will be at first little or no movement and you will have to work on freeing this area.

Everyone, and I mean everyone, has felt something in their back at some time. It may just be a dull ache after a lot of bending or sitting, or it may be acute pain from disc problems. Whatever your level of problem I would urge you not to give up and use your back as an excuse to do nothing. If you stop using it, it will seize up, so simple gentle movements are essential. If you are under treatment always check with your doctor or therapist, but don't be satisfied by an overworked doctor who prescribes pain killers and tells you nebulously to 'be careful' because he hasn't got time to explain. There are several good books which deal with back problems and how to lie down, sit, stand, and carry things. Read them and act on them. The longer you allow the back to seize up, the more permanent that seizing up becomes. Keep mobile, keep moving. I will give you exercises to help with this. Sometimes they are uncomfortable at first but keep trying, don't give up. Exercise does work! Don't *ever* try to start at the strongest level of exercise because you think that you will get there quicker. All that happens is that you overdo it and you will have to start from the beginning again or, worse still, you will damage yourself. Do little and often! Remember too that *pain* is a warning sign and although you should feel your body working, and this feeling can be strong, sharp pains mean stop – IMMEDIATELY!

BUTTOCKS SQUEEZE (Chart Ex. 18)

Let's start by finding those gluteal muscles and getting a bit of life back into them! Sitting on your hard stool or chair with your back upright, clench your buttocks together and then release. And again, and again, so you are bobbing up and down. Well perhaps you're not; sometimes it is a bit difficult to locate those muscles at first, so try pressing down with your thighs and pushing on the outside of your feet. Look for a ripple or a stir in the side of your bottom and then build it into a dimple.

Now you've got your buttocks dimpling in – I love this exercise, it is my all time favourite – what else can you feel? Depending on the amount of flesh on your bottom it could be anything from a bounce to a crunch of sitting bones each time you let go (remember the sitting bones from your correct sitting?) If this is the case, tilt your pelvis by pulling in your tummy (the top half stays in the same place so you're not leaning back) and then you will loose the sitting bones every time you land, which makes it more comfortable.

Another thing you might feel is a tightening of the inside thigh – you see you cannot truly separate one bit from another. Everything you do has a consequence somewhere else; what we are trying to do is to get you pulled together in a positive way so everything is working in harmony and balance.

BUTTOCKS SQUEEZE WITH LEGS RAISED (Chart Ex. 19)

When you have mastered the basic squeeze try bringing in the tummy muscles too. Fold your arms to give you a forward balance – do this without rounding your shoulders round your ears. Tilt your pelvis by pulling your tummy muscles in. Don't lean back, just tilt back as you practised in the correct sitting. Stretch your legs out in front of you and let them roll outwards, resting your feet on the floor. Keep your tummy muscles pulled in all the time because now your legs are forward you are working on your tummy too. While your tummy muscles are pulled in and your pelvis tilted, your back is released. If your tummy is too weak to hold this or you feel anything in your back, leave this stage until you are stronger. If everything feels okay, then squeeze and release your buttocks. Once you've got this going try varying the speed, some slower ones to get deeper into the muscle (don't overdo this and hold for too long) and some really quick ones for the surface muscles.

One thing to watch for! Make sure it is your buttocks doing the work and that you are not doing all the work with your shoulders

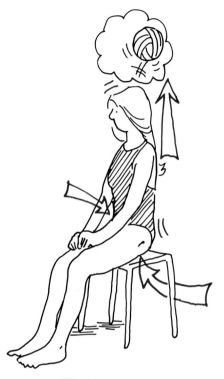

The buttocks squeeze

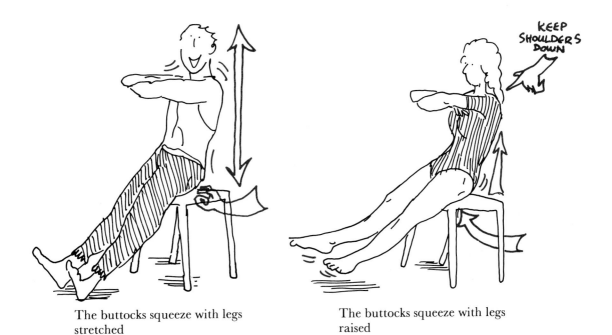

The buttocks squeeze with legs stretched

The buttocks squeeze with legs raised

and the centre of your body. If this is the case, go back to the first stage and get the muscles really working before you try again.

The next stage is to lift your legs off the ground, keeping them straight and turned out with your feet relaxed at the end. Now you are holding the weight of your legs with your tummy muscles, so it is even more important to keep them pulled in to protect your back. Squeeze away until you feel a wonderful glow. I particularly like doing this one to music.

If your job involves a lot of sitting then your buttocks are being stretched all that time. No wonder they spread and get flabby. I would like to see all sitting workers, from lorry drivers to typists to the boss, squeezing their buttocks at least twice a day. I always want to smile when I do this exercise, and I'm sure everyone would have happier days and lovelier bottoms if they squeezed while they worked!

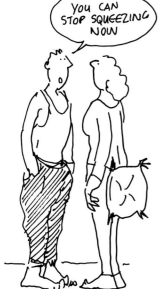

BRIDGE LIFT (Chart Ex. 41)

The next exercise might cause a bit more of a stir around the office, so I recommend it for home use only. Lie on your back and put your feet flat on the floor with your knees bent. Now tilt your pelvis by pulling in your tummy. If you have problems with this, skip ahead to the next chapter for full details of the pelvic tilt lying down. As your tummy muscles pull in, your pubic bone moves up and forwards and your back releases. Now push your lifted pubic bone upwards until your back lifts off the floor in a

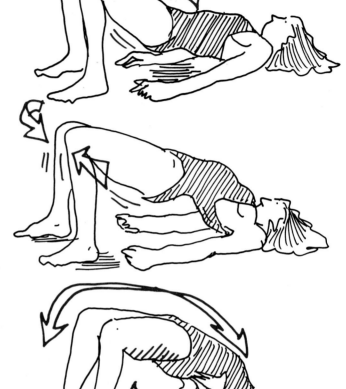

The bridge lift –
1. Push up pubic bone until bridge is formed.

2. Pushing up and squeezing thighs and buttocks together.

3. Heels off ground, back supported by hands to get further lift.

bridge position. Place your hands in the small of your back with your thumbs on the outside so that the hands are supporting your back. Lift your heels off the floor so you are resting on the balls of your feet and move your feet in a little closer if you need to. Not too close, or you'll collapse. Get the maximum lift you can without 'squeezing' your lower back – try to get your elbows underneath you and your heels on the floor. If you're very weak or not too mobile, hold this position for a few minutes or as long as you can. Any pain in the small of your back means you should come straight out of it.

To lower yourself down, reverse the way you got up there. Ripple down through your back, vertebra by vertebra, from the shoulders down through the tilt of your pelvis, tummy muscles in and helping to control your descent. Bending your knees into your chest will release your back after this exercise but you can usually try it a couple of times before you do that. Bending your knees into your chest also gives a good indication of how tight your lower back is. If your knees won't come into your chest or will only come in if your bottom tips up off the floor, then your lower back is tight. This position and 'the ball', described later, will help release it.

As soon as this basic lift presents no problems, the second stage can be attempted. This involves getting into the basic lift position and holding it without the hands (they are resting on the floor beside you); with your heels down release a little of the lift, then squeeze your buttocks and thrust upwards. Keep going, releasing and squeezing until your buttocks glow. Come down slowly and pull in your knees as before.

The third stage brings in the inside thigh as well. Exactly the same action as in the previous stage but as you thrust upwards bring your inside thighs together. Really squeeze everything inwards. You'll feel it in the tops of your thighs too at first (this should produce a glow). Don't forget to pull your knees in at the end to release your back.

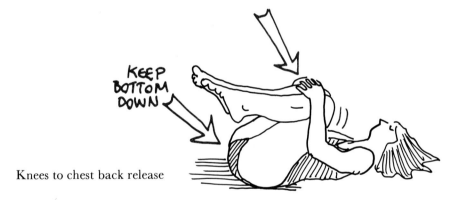

KEEP BOTTOM DOWN

Knees to chest back release

Let's now move on to the back muscles themselves. The important ones to deal with first are the *erector spinae*. These are the muscles that run on either side of the spine, supporting it and helping the ligaments hold it in place. They should be prominent on either side of the spine, leaving a groove down the centre of your back. The best way to get into them is by lifting your legs and the top half of your body while lying on your tummy; but nothing is quite as simple as that, so here are the whys and hows.

We'll start with leg lifts. Lie down on your tummy. If you have very prominent hip bones or a weak back or just want to make this more comfortable, put a cushion under your pelvis at waist level and below. This will gently lift the pelvis and take the pressure off the curve of your spine.

Place one hand on top of the other and rest your forehead on your hands. This is important as it will keep your neck long and

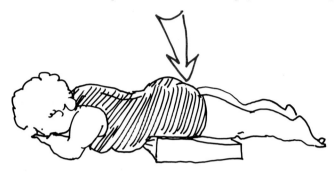

Strengthening the back muscles – starting position

released. If your chin was on your hands, your neck would shorten and this could build up tension. Make sure that the weight of your body is on your chest and not on your elbows. If you try to help your legs by pushing up with your elbows, you will build up the tension in your shoulders.

I am starting with the most simple leg lift. This is for people with very weak backs and can be bypassed by most people. It is very important, though, however weak your back, that you should try to strengthen it. Otherwise you could end up totally debilitated.

When you lift your leg or legs up behind you they act as weights. You can alter the amount of weight you use by changing the length of your leg. If you lift your leg with the knee bent, you are lifting less weight than you would be if your leg was straight. This is the law of levers after all. We do have similarities to mechanical devices!

LEG LIFTS (Chart Ex. 42)

So for your first steps towards strengthening a weak back bend your knees in and lift *one* leg at a time alternately, very slowly and gently trying to keep your hips down. Don't tire yourself but don't give up. You will get the strength back in those muscles.

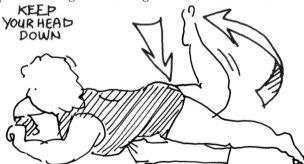

Leg lifts – one leg at a time, bend your knee to lessen weight

Back to the mechanics again. What should be happening here is that the buttocks squeeze in to lift the legs upwards. The back muscles also contract and shorten as the leg lifts into the back.

The more a muscle is worked, the more it comes back to life. I must emphasise again that when contracting a muscle it is more beneficial to contract and release than to hold the contraction for a long time. Do not, when lifting your leg or legs, try to bypass the buttocks and lift on the back muscles alone. It will put too much strain on them and that is what your buttocks are there for – *to support your back*. I hope this is beginning to come together and make sense to you.

Okay, so your back's stronger now or it wasn't that bad in the first place, but it's still on the weak side. The next stage to try is straight single leg raises.

With your legs straight out behind you – no bent knees this time – squeeze your buttocks together and lift one leg at a time alternately. Don't go on relentlessly, start with two lifts with each leg then a rest and then two more and build up. But don't try to hold for too long. Make each lift deliberate and controlled, bringing the leg up and down at an even pace and don't lift your hip.

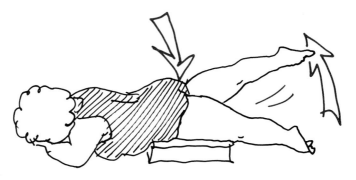

Leg lifts – one at a time, straight leg adds weight

We next bring in both legs. Now you really have increased the weight of your lever so it becomes even more important not to bypass the buttocks when you lift.

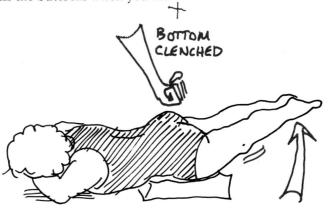

Leg lifts with both legs straight

Keep your legs and feet together, don't let them splay apart, and clench your buttocks together. Raise the legs up and lower them. Try a set of four, then rest. If your top half hovers off the ground as you lift your legs (which it shouldn't do if you are using a cushion), relax it down and take the lift more gently. When you rest between sets of lifts turn your head to the side and take a deep breath to help you release, turning it to a different side after each set. Aim to get the front of your thighs off the ground, with your legs straight.

When you have finished your leg lifts it is very important that you stretch out the back muscles again so you don't get negative tension building up.

THE BALL POSITION (Chart Ex. 49)

This is the ball position: come up on to your knees, push away the cushion, sit back on your heels, then fold your body forwards over your thighs. Tuck your head in and rest your arms back along your legs with your palms turned upwards by your feet. This

The ball position – stretching entire length of spine

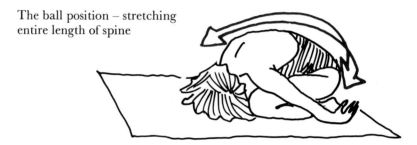

stretches right through your spine from the base through to the back of the neck. It should feel wonderful. If, however, this feels claustrophobic or you have sinus trouble and it puts pressure in your head, try stretching your arms out in front of you and just resting your forehead on the ground in front of you like a cat stretching. This should be very restful.

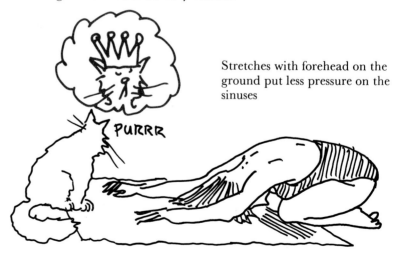

Stretches with forehead on the ground put less pressure on the sinuses

PURRR

SOME HARDER EXERCISES

These are only to be tried when your back is really strong enough and copes well with the first ones. Back into the same position with or without the cushion (a towel or rug can be sufficient if your hip bones are the problem).

LEG LIFT VARIATIONS (Chart Ex. 42)

Straight leg lift in a set of four, but keeping the feet off the floor all the time so that you get no complete release in between. Lift and halfway down, lift and halfway down, etc.

LEG LIFTS WITH LEGS APART (Chart Ex. 43)

A variation is to do leg lifts with the legs apart. Lift up the legs and exaggerate the outward movement, then lower with the legs still apart (no bent knees and thighs off the ground). This can also be done without putting the legs on the floor each time.

LEGS UP AND APART IN THE AIR (Chart Ex. 44)

This combines the straight leg lift and the legs apart. Lift your legs up, hold them there, then take them apart and bring them together (this is good for the inside thigh too). Finish by bringing them together and lowering them to the floor.

Legs up together, apart and down

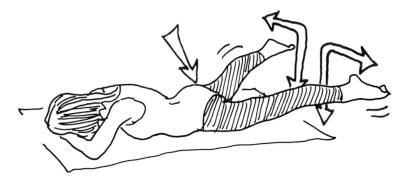

LEGS UP TOGETHER, APART AND DOWN (Chart Ex. 45)

Lift the legs up together, then take them apart as far as they will go; bring them together again, still in the air, then lower them. Keep this as smooth as possible and don't jerk them up and out and in and down.

LEG CIRCLES (Chart Ex. 46)

This is a hard exercise. Take your legs apart and lift them up. Keep them straight and then make small inward and outward circles from the *thigh*. For outward circles exaggerate the upward and outward movement, for inward circles exaggerate the outward and then the upward movement. Try four of each slowly at first, then build up and vary the pace.

Leg circles with movements made
from thigh

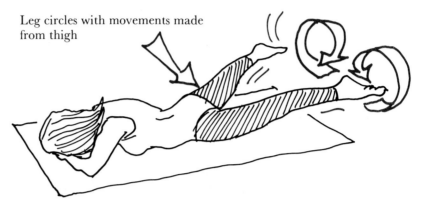

In all exercise it is important to use control. This is not easy at first, but aim for it because once you have control of your movement you are master or mistress of your body and *you* can decide what you want to do and not make your body an excuse.

Do go easy at first on the back exercises and build up sensibly and *remember* to squeeze your buttocks before you lift your legs. This is only a book and I cannot be there to see you do it. Give your legs a rest for a while. Next we'll bring in another weight and lever: the top half of your body. (Sorry, but the cushion has to go now as it won't be of any further help.)

ARM LIFTS (Chart Ex. 47)

Straighten your arms out in front of you. If you are very weak, raise one arm at a time lifting your head and looking up. The next stage is to lift both arms together with the top part of your body. Try linking your thumbs together to stop your arms splaying

Arm lifts, both arms together

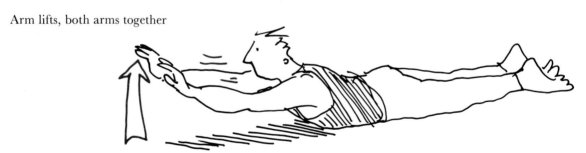

apart. It helps if you breathe in as you lift up. It doesn't matter if you only come a little way off the ground – you are still working the muscles.

ARM AND LEG LIFTS TOGETHER (Chart Ex. 48)

Putting the two halves together: when you feel you are strong enough to try both halves together, start with one arm and one leg at a time. Make these opposite arm to leg so as not to put too much strain on one side of the body. Lift your right arm and your left leg, then your left arm and your right leg. Don't forget to look up along your arm as you lift.

Arm and leg lifts together – lifting opposite arm and leg

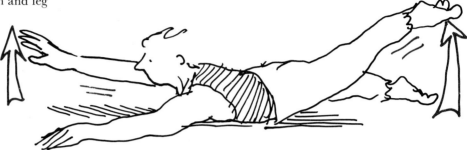

When you've got that working well, try both arms and legs. There are two ways you can do this: the easiest way is by clasping your hands behind you, straightening your arms and using them to help 'pull' the top half of you up and back, at the same time squeezing your buttocks and lifting your legs; the slightly harder version is with the arms out full stretch in front of you, maximum lever weight.

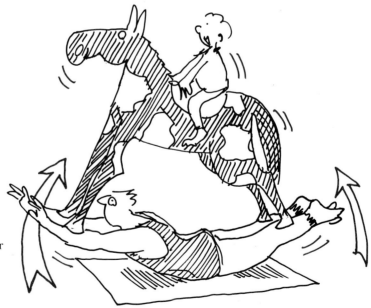

Arms and legs lifts, both together with maximum lever weight

Don't forget your ball position when you've finished; it is very important. Or go into it halfway through your back exercises just to give yourself a break.

CAT STRETCH (Chart Ex. 50)

When you come out of your ball position try a moving release for your back on your hands and knees. Your arms should be straight down from your shoulders and your legs straight down from your hips; pull in your tummy (yes, this is yet another way of doing

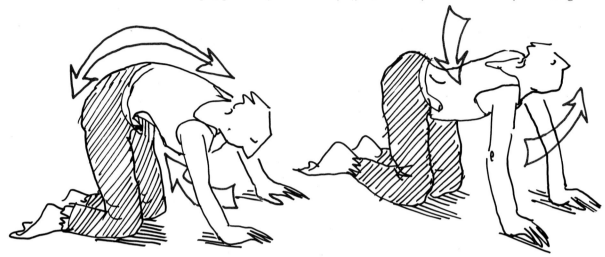

Cat stretch to release – back rounded, tummy in   Cat stretch – back arched, head lifted

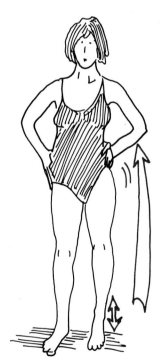

The sideways pelvic tilt, standing with feet slightly apart

the pelvic tilt) so that your back rounds, then release and let your back arch. Your head should follow the movement. As you pull in your tummy and round your back your head drops down, and as your back arches your head drops back. If your back is already overarched and/or weak don't go into a full arch, just come back to the flat back position with your head straight forward.

Here is another exercise I would like to recommend for releasing the back.

THE SIDEWAYS PELVIC TILT (Chart Ex. 57)

Try this exercise lying down at first. Flat on your back, stretch out your right leg until your left hip comes up, then your left leg until your right hip comes up; keep going first one side, then the other. You can either do this on the floor or in bed when you get the aches. To do the sideways tilt standing up, stand with your feet slightly apart and then left your right hip and heel and then lift your left hip and heel. Each time the hip lifts, your waist muscles shorten so you're helping them too. If you put your hand on your lower back you can actually feel the muscles working and releasing.

BENT KNEE ROLLING (Chart Ex. 58)

Twisting also releases and mobilises the spine. This twist is done lying on your back using your bent legs as weights, so don't try it if your back is weak. Lie flat on your back with your arms out on either side of you at shoulder level, palms pressed into the floor. Bend your knees into your chest and then roll them slowly from side to side keeping them pressed together. Keep your shoulders down on the ground. To rotate right through the spine, roll your head in the opposite direction to your legs so your head is going to the right as your legs go to the left and then everything comes to the centre before your head goes to the left and your legs to the right. Not only does this help loosen your spine but your tummy muscles are helping to lift your legs from side to side. To understand this better we must go into the next chapter.

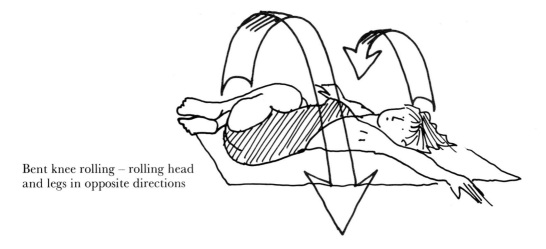

Bent knee rolling – rolling head and legs in opposite directions

Recommended books for further information on backs:

Avoiding Back Trouble published by the Consumers' Association London, 1978

You are as young as your spine by Editha Hearn published by Heinemann, London, 1975

Both explain very simply about slipped discs and give practical advice on how to cope with your problem.

5 The 'Abdominals', Pelvic Tilt and The 'Rude' Bits

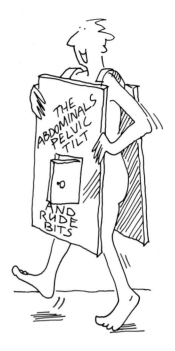

The abdominals are the lifetime girdle, or at least that's what their designer intended. But through lack of proper use the elastic goes slack and everything starts to drop and bulge out. Fortunately muscles, unlike elastic, can be revitalised.

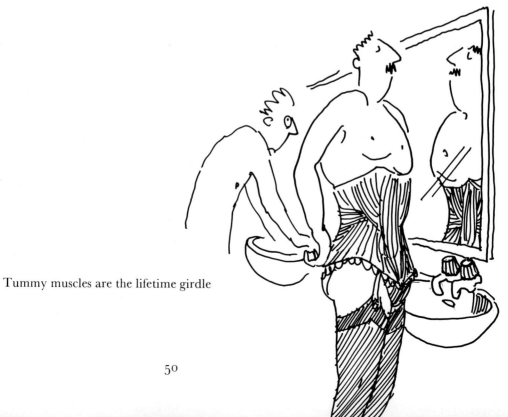

Tummy muscles are the lifetime girdle

The abdominals

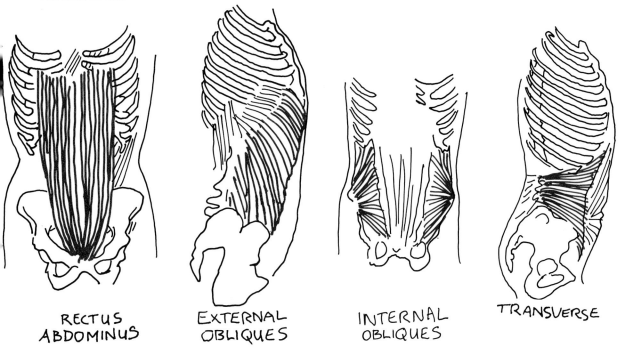

RECTUS ABDOMINUS

EXTERNAL OBLIQUES

INTERNAL OBLIQUES

TRANSVERSE

Pregnant woman and husband with beer paunch: back muscles no longer able to cope with extra weight pulling forwards – result, backache

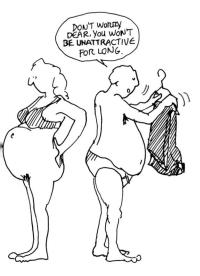

DON'T WORRY DEAR. YOU WON'T BE UNATTRACTIVE FOR LONG.

Let's start by having a look at the structure of this large muscle group. First, there are the *rectus* muscles which run up and down the front of the body on either side of a ligament, called the *linea alba*, which attaches to the breast bone at the top and the pubic bone of the pelvis below. Then there are the internal and external obliques, muscles which run in layers, one above the other, diagonally across the body. Lastly, there is the deepest layer of muscles which run from side to side and are called the transverse muscles.

Between them, this criss-cross arrangement of muscles controls an enormous range of movements and the state of our posture. Yet even when they have been allowed to weaken we don't collapse in a heap. So where is the work being done? Have a look at the illustration showing two familiar and similar shapes. Notice the two compensatory curves and there's your answer. When the tummy muscles protrude, the extra weight is forced into the back muscles. When these can no longer cope and too much pressure is put on the spine, the result is backache and eventually this can lead to disc damage and severe pain.

One third of the spine is made up of intervertebral discs. These are cartilaginous shock absorbers which separate the vertebrae. These discs are made up of two flat layers held together by an outer band. Contained within this structure is a gelatinous substance which can ooze around as pressure is moved from one side

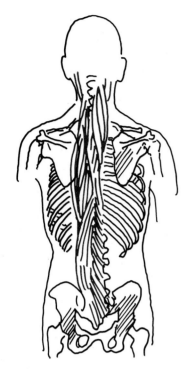

Showing the spine held in place by two ligaments and by the *erector spinae* muscles

to the other. This allows the spine its wonderful range of articulation. The spine is held in place by two ligaments (ligaments are thick fibrous bands which hold a joint in place, unlike muscles which are elastic and which move the joints as well as helping keep them firm) and by the *erector spinae* muscles which are equivalent to the *rectus abdominus*. These are the muscles which form the groove down the back on either side of the spine. They are the muscles which we strengthened by lifting the legs up behind in the last chapter. (If there is no groove down your back, keep working on those muscles to build them up!)

You may be wondering why I didn't deal with all this in the last chapter, when I was talking about backs! It is actually very hard to separate backs and fronts since some of the tummy muscles and the hip flexors, which I am coming to, all attach to the spine and this makes the action of one integral with the other's. Muscles have to work in pairs in order to move a joint. When you pull your tummy muscles and round your back the tummy muscles are shortening whilst the back muscles are releasing. This is extremely important to remember while you perform tummy muscle exercises. So many people do tummy muscle exercises which are *far* too strong for them or do them wrongly and complain afterwards that all they can feel is a pain in their back!

And this is where the hidden danger comes in – the hip flexors. You can't see these muscles since they are situated inside you, so when they are working there is no external ripple; you just feel them pull on your back when you overuse them. They attach to the lower lumbar vertebrae, run down through the pelvis, then divide off and attach to the head of each of your thigh bones (femurs). Their action is to flex your hips and you use them every time you walk, so they are usually well exercised. They will also take over the job of the abdominals when they are too weak in trunk and leg raising exercises.

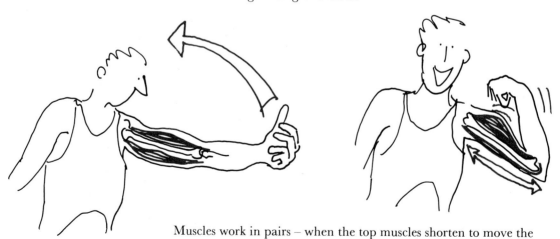

Muscles work in pairs – when the top muscles shorten to move the lower arm up, the underneath muscles must lengthen to allow the movement

Two of the most popular tummy muscle exercises given are sit-ups and double leg raising. If your tummy muscles are not strong enough, both these movements can be done by the hip flexors with the back arched and the tummy muscles bulging and stretching. Yes, *stretching*, which makes their weakness worse!

When I had my baby in hospital in 1970 I was given double leg raising as a tummy muscle exercise – the very worst possible thing when the tummy muscles are at their weakest! Unfortunately I did not know then what I know now, otherwise I would have been able to take responsibility for my own body and not given myself awful backache by performing this totally unsuitable exercise.

I am including all this simple anatomy in the hope that you will understand the basics of how your body works and why certain exercises should only be done when sufficient strength has already been developed. This applies to men as well as women even though their muscles are naturally stronger. It is *your* body and, ultimately, its care is your responsibility. *You* are the one who will suffer if something goes wrong.

I am not trying to put you off building up to strong exercises or ever doing anything in case you hurt yourself. Feeling your muscles work is feeling you are alive! I love the feeling of muscles glowing and the wonderful energy you release when you have really worked your body. But there is a great difference between *keeping* fit and *getting* fit, so take it in stages and remember that acute pain is a warning sign.

Before we start to exercise the tummy just go back to thinking about your image in the mirror. The more slumped you are the more your tummy pushes out. So why is it such an effort not to slouch? Because the tummy muscles are weak! The old vicious circle. The trunk contains two bony structures, the ribs and the

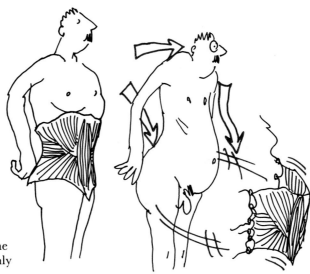

Showing the space between the ribs and the pelvis which is only supported by muscle

pelvis, but between these there is a space which is only supported by muscles. When these muscles are weak the ribs collapse down towards the pelvis and the result is that the centre concertinas and pushes out! The slump also has an effect on the spine. Remember the spine is one third spongey discs. Pressure on these can cause them to squash down and you can measurably shrink nearly a quarter of an inch in a day! When you sleep and the pressure is taken off the discs, they gradually come back to normal again. As we age, though, they begin to loose their springiness so it becomes doubly important not to slump. Slumping and other pressures on the spine as well as knocks and jars can cause weaknesses in the outer band of the disc so that some of the jelly substance inside pushes out unevenly. This causes the disc to become lopsided or prolapsed so that one vertebra pushes down on to the other, pinching the nerves which run out between them. This is what we call a slipped disc. Very often the disc will pop back into place naturally but meanwhile the muscles surrounding it will have gone into spasm to create a protective splint. This is the cause of much back pain. Discs don't just suddenly pop out. There is a long build up of weakness before some very small movement proves to be the final straw. So it *does* matter how you sit and stand; it's not just vanity.

I think a bit of vanity *is* important, too. We should take a pride in our appearance and how we present ourselves. Holding yourself well should not be such an effort and it immediately makes you look and feel better.

There are some people who look really thin but still complain about their tummies. Every muscle in our bodies is covered by a layer of fat but the tummy muscles have two layers of fat, one on either side of the muscle. Women have a thicker fat layer than men, which gives them their rounded, more feminine shape; this applies to tummies too. A man with a good physique should have a groove

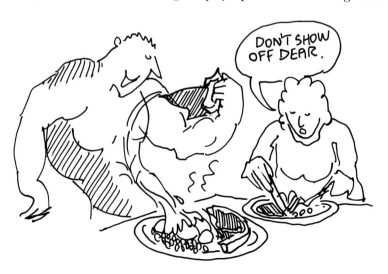

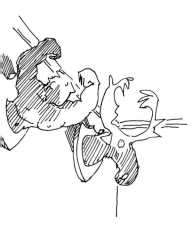

down the centre of his body. These are the *rectus abdominis* muscles pulling into their central ligament (like the *erector spinae* pulling into the spine at the back). In women there should be the same muscle definition, but softer and less pronounced – unless you wish to develop a body builder's physique. The body builder's physique is the result of a combination of extremely strong weight training (and this should reassure anyone who thinks that exercise might overdevelop muscle), strict diet and dietary supplements. The result is that all the body fat is burned off and is replaced by muscle bulk.

I know you are dying to get on with some exercises, but I want this book to help you understand your body so that whatever you do, you will do it properly. So please bear with me a little longer.

During your lifetime certain muscles will just go on working away without a passing thought from you. You may be conscious of the in- and out-goings of your food, but not of what goes on in between – the same with your heart and your breathing – yet the functions of these involuntary muscles are vital to life. Let's have a quick look at how they lie and how external exercises can affect them.

The trunk is divided into two chambers: the thorax (chest) and abdomen (tummy area). The divider is a dome-shaped muscle called the diaphragm. This has a central ligament and attaches all round to the side of the trunk. Above the diaphragm we find the heart and lungs and below the diaphragm, still under the protective umbrella of the ribs, are the liver, stomach, spleen and kidneys. Then, unprotected by any bony structures, fall the coils of intestines where the goodness from our food is absorbed and the rest is prepared for elimination. The lower part of the intestines, the bladder and the reproductive organs are then contained in the pelvic basin.

In order to breathe, the chest cavity is kept at a minus pressure. This means that if you were punctured in the chest it would all cave in. On the other hand the abdomen is kept at plus pressure, which helps us eliminate waste food and liquid and bear down in child birth. If you were punctured in the abdomen everything would burst out.

To understand the significance of these two pressures let's first look at the breathing mechanism. In order to breathe 'in' the chest must expand. This draws air down into the lungs. To expand the chest the ribs and diaphragm work together. The diaphragm flattens downwards and at the same time the ribs lift upwards and outwards, sucking in air. This is active breathing. Breathing out is passive as the diaphragm relaxes and comes back to its dome shape and the ribs fall back into place.

Try putting your hands on your ribs to feel this action. Many people lose the use of the muscles between the ribs by continual shallow breathing, so that the ribs eventually become fixed. Be

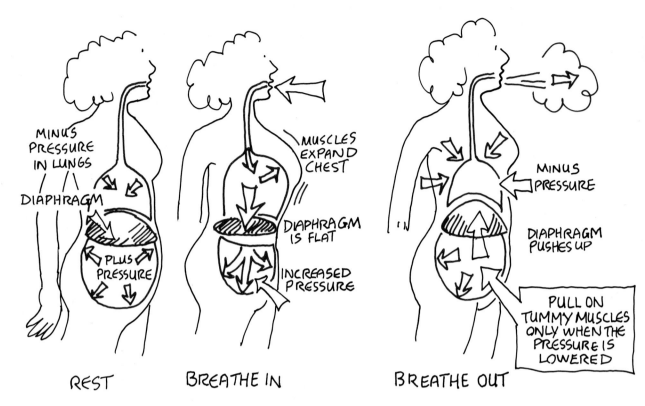

MINUS PRESSURE IN LUNGS

DIAPHRAGM

PLUS PRESSURE

REST

MUSCLES EXPAND CHEST

DIAPHRAGM IS FLAT

INCREASED PRESSURE

BREATHE IN

MINUS PRESSURE

DIAPHRAGM PUSHES UP

PULL ON TUMMY MUSCLES ONLY WHEN THE PRESSURE IS LOWERED

BREATHE OUT

The breathing mechanism – active and passive breathing

careful not to take too many deep breaths while practising this movement, otherwise you may feel dizzy and eventually faint!

When the diaphragm flattens with the in breath, it takes up space in the abdominal cavity. This causes the already plus pressure to rise and is why the tummy expands slightly during normal breathing.

What on earth has all this got to do with my tummy muscles, you are now wondering! Well, would you fill a balloon up with air and squeeze it? Not unless you wanted it to pop! And yet how often have you breathed in and pulled in your tummy muscles to zip up too tight jeans or squeeze through a narrow space?

Think again: when you breathe in you push *up* the abdominal pressure, so pulling in the tummy muscles should coincide with the *out* breath. Holding your breath can be just as bad, as this will also increase the pressure. I have often seen people with bright red faces and pursed lips concentrating on what they are doing and holding their breath fiercely so that they are left gasping at the end of an exercise. The result can be more dangerous. Pushing up the pressure affects your heart as well as the abdominal organs.

These are contained in a sack called the peritoneum. If the wall of the peritoneum is weakened and too much pressure is applied, the result is a hernia. This means that part of the intestines rupture the peritoneum and burst through. Many hernias are caused by pushing and lifting heavy objects while holding the breath. This also puts pressure on the pelvic floor.

Understanding the theory behind breathing out with a tummy muscles contraction is often easier than putting it into practice. This has to be learned and we will start very simply with the pelvic tilt. Whatever exercise you are doing, though, try to breathe with it rhythmically so that your whole body works together.

THE PELVIC TILT (Chart Ex. 9)

Simple, safe and effective for all! Lie on your back and bend your knees up so that your feet are flat on the ground. Put your hands on your tummy at first so that you can feel what's happening.

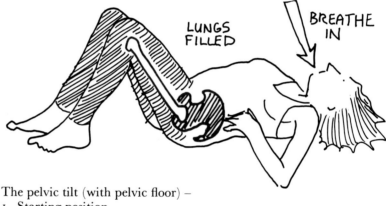

The pelvic tilt (with pelvic floor) –
1. Starting position

(Breathe in deeply so that when you contract your abdominal muscles you've got to breathe out!)

Pull your tummy muscles down (contract) so that your back presses into the floor. As the tummy muscles shorten they pull on the pubic bone, tipping it up towards your head. This should leave a scooped-out basin in the centre of your body. No, your back should not come off the floor – try again. Sometimes even the simplest movements take time to master. Also, if your back is very tight this will restrict the movement. Remember that as the tummy muscles shorten the back will release. That's why this exercise is particularly good for starting you off and for maintaining muscle movement, however weak you are.

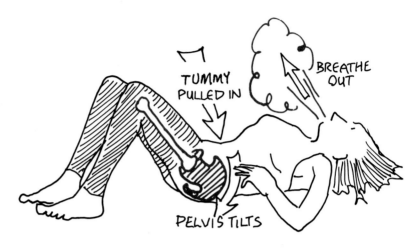

2. Breathing out and pulling in the tummy

To stretch your back, bend your knees and clasp your hands round them and then pull them into your chest, *without* your

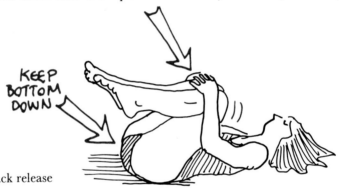

Knees to chest back release

bottom moving up off the floor; then there is no problem with the tightness of your back muscles. If the knees won't go down into your chest or your bottom rolls up off the ground, then your back needs stretching out. So more slow, gentle knee to chest squeezes, or try the 'ball' position. The more you work these muscles, the more they will free; so do some back leg lifts as well with plenty of release afterwards (as described in the last chapter).

By extending the breathing with the pelvic tilt you can increase its strength enormously. So much so that if you have a contraceptive coil it could dislodge it. Therefore use your discretion about trying this exercise.

Breathe in deeply. Start breathing out slowly and tilt your pelvis (make sure you can do this properly before you try this stronger version). Go on breathing out until you feel as if there is no air left in your body (of course there is some left as you haven't breathed your last breath yet!). No more air left to breathe out?

58

Right – now suck in your tummy as far as you can. With very little air in your body and the pressure down, your tummy muscles will pull into the vacuum leaving you with a great dent in the middle and right up under your ribs. Hold this as long as you can so that when you feel you can't hold any longer you gasp the air back in. Not only will this work on your tummy muscles but it also has the effect of gently massaging your bowels which aids your digestion and can also be helpful if you are a bit constipated (it won't give you diarrhoea). It is also important to see that the more you breathe out the more you can pull in.

NOSE TO TOES (Chart Ex. 31)

You don't need to do vast movements and puff and groan to make your muscles work effectively. Lie on your back and put your hands on your tummy so that you can feel the muscles shortening.

Nose to toes

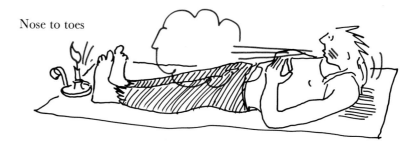

Now all you have to do is lift your head – chin to chest – and flex your toes up towards you at the same time. Those two small inward movements are enough to contract your tummy muscles effectively. Practise the breathing. Always breathe in first, then breathe out as you flex your toes and look at them.

CURL-UPS (Chart Ex. 30)

As soon as you add a bit of body weight against the pull of gravity of course, the muscles will have to work that much harder. So, still lying on your back, bend your knees up again and put your feet flat on the floor. Breathe in. Breathe out and pull down on your tummy muscles pressing your lower back into the floor and lift your head and shoulders up and forward, stretching your arms out towards your knees. Breathe in as you come down. Try to get both the movement and the breathing rhythmical rather than jerking yourself up, holding it for a second and then flopping flat on the floor. The same with the breathing: don't gasp a quick breath in, hold it and then breathe it all out at once! Try to control both all the way through.

So far you haven't lifted your lower back off the floor, so that it has been protected. Before you do try lifting the back off the floor, lessen the help from your arms by first of all folding them and then placing them behind your head as you perform the same movements. So –

Stage 1. Curl-up with arms straight forwards

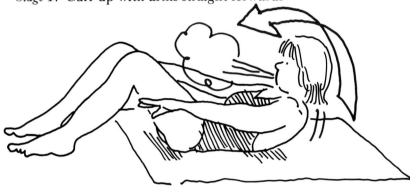

Stage 2. Curl-ups with folded arms

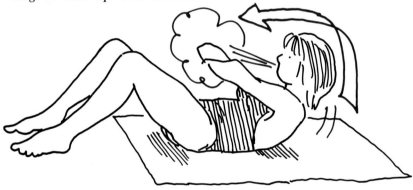

Stage 3. Curl-ups with the hands behind the head

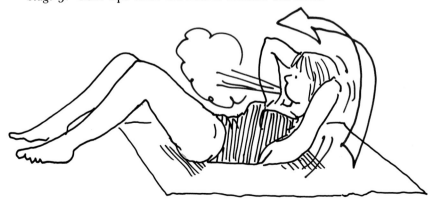

Always start with stage 1 and then when you know the tummy muscles are really working go on to the next stages. Never quiver or over-strain in an exercise.

You may find that as you do this exercise you begin to feel it more in your neck than in your tummy, especially if your neck is already overtight. Feeling a pull in the front of the neck is quite a good exercise for the front neck muscles, so don't worry about this. If the back of the neck is the problem, it is important not to allow too much negative tension to build up – just do a set of four curl-ups, then have a rest. While you are resting roll your head from side to side keeping it supported on the floor.

You can vary the speed of your curl-ups. Try some slow ones for more control, then some quick ones to get you going.

Up to now we have worked mostly on the up-and-down front tummy muscles (the *rectus* muscles) but it is important to bring in the obliques also. The same curl-up can be used, but this time you twist and pull over to one side at a time. Try this in the same three stages.

Stage 1. Straight arms pull first to the right side of the knees, while turning the right shoulder back to twist the chest round. Push down onto the right hip and then twist and pull to the left in the same way. Don't forget the breathing.

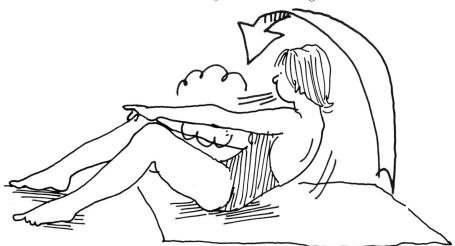

Curl-up with diagonal twist: arms straight, knees bent

Stage 2. The same twisting and lifting movement but with folded arms.

Curl-up with diagonal twist:
arms folded, knees bent

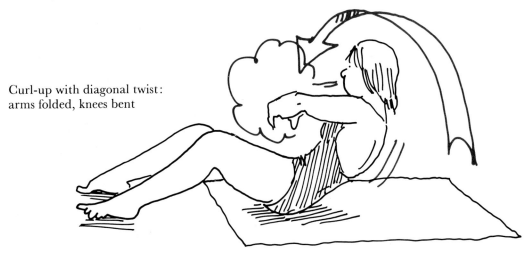

NOW TRY WITH HANDS
BEHIND YOUR HEAD

Stage 3. As stage 2, but with the hands behind your head.

The most important thing is to keep your back rounded so that you are working on the tummy muscles. As soon as you try to straighten your back you are bringing in the hip flexors.

CONTRACTIONS (Chart Ex. 32)

These are similar to the curl-ups, but you start with the legs straight. Flex your toes up towards you (keeping the heels on the floor) and slightly bend your knees. At the same time try and lift the top half of your body keeping the back slightly curved. Bend your arms and push forwards with the heel of your hand. This will help you to lift your body up. Keep your head back – try looking up – to stop it poking forward and straining your neck. This is harder than the curl-ups, so start by just lifting the top half of the body from the floor – tummy contracted in, lower back pressed in the floor and breathing out. Come up to the centre then to the right, then to the left. When your tummy muscles are really strong you will be able to come right up. Try slow ones – four counts up and four counts down – for control, and try quick ones too to get right into the muscle.

CURL-DOWNS (Chart Ex. 56)

These can be used as an alternative to curl-ups and they don't affect the neck. It is a sort of reverse sit-up. Start by sitting on the floor with your legs out in front of you. Fold your arms to add a balancing weight in front of you, but don't hunch your shoulders.

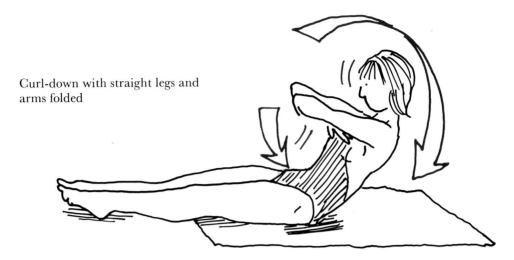

Curl-down with straight legs and arms folded

From sitting up straight pull your tummy muscles in enough to tilt your pelvis back. Don't go any further until you've got that first contraction. Now your tummy muscles are pulled in and strong, start to slowly *curl* your body downwards until you feel its weight held by your tummy muscles. If the muscles start to quiver or bulge, you have gone too far. Holding your curled position, bring your body back up, then straighten your back into your starting position. The beauty of this exercise is that you are in control all the time because you have started from your point of strength, unlike the sit-up where you are starting from your weakest point. As the muscles strengthen you will be able to curl down further without them quivering or bulging. Quivering is the first sign that they are losing their grip. Bulging is when they start stretching and the hip flexors begin to take over. Make sure you keep your shoulders relaxed and remember to breathe out as you curl downwards, in as you come up.

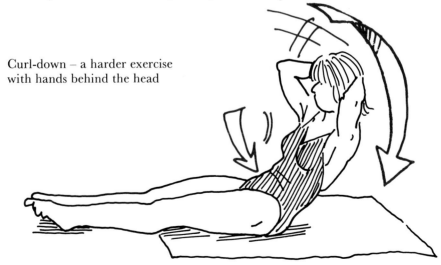

Curl-down – a harder exercise with hands behind the head

You can make this exercise harder by putting your hands behind your head, but make sure you know what you're doing first.

If you can get down to the floor and curl up again, you have then worked up to a correct sit-up. These should always be done with a slightly curled back – a straight back involves too much use of the hip flexors – and they should be performed with the feet free. In other words, if you can't get up without someone

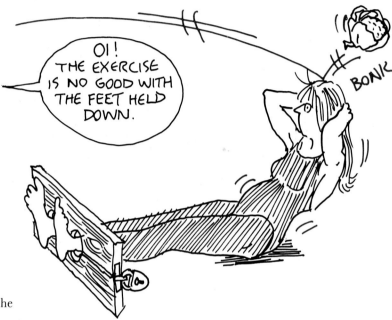

OI! THE EXERCISE IS NO GOOD WITH THE FEET HELD DOWN.

BONK

Curl-down – should be with the feet free

holding your feet or sticking them under a chair, your tummy muscles still aren't strong enough to do this exercise. Sit-ups are an advanced exercise for athletic training and are not necessary for getting your tummy muscles into good shape.

A word of warning here. If you have had major abdominal surgery or if your abdominal muscles have separated during pregnancy, you must grade your tummy muscle exercises gradually afterwards. Always check with your doctor or physiotherapist first if you are not sure. Exercise is very important however bad the muscles are but do make sure you are doing one which is beneficial to you. Separation in pregnancy is when the rectus muscles 'separate' from the central ligament; you can actually feel this with your fingers. Normally these muscles will nearly always pull together again with time, but do go to ante- and post-natal classes. If the weakening is permanent, you must keep exercising gently.

There are many variations of trunk raising exercises. Having given you the inside facts on 'why' and some examples of 'how', I do hope that you will be able to get the most out of any other versions you are given from now on. The same applies to tummy exercises using the legs, which we will have a look at now.

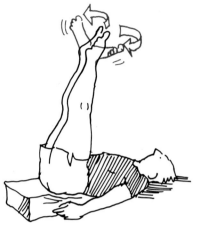

Legs in the air – resting position

SINGLE LEG LOWERING (Chart Ex. 36)

Start by bending your knees into your chest, then lift into the air. This is your resting position! With the legs straight up in the air, the pull of gravity should run through the centre of them so that there is no resistance in any direction. As soon as they move down and away from you, the weight of your legs and the pull of gravity will come into force. If your hamstring muscles at the back of your thighs are very tight and your legs rather weak, trying to hold your legs in the resting position can be anything but restful! To help you with this, put a cushion underneath you at waist level and below. This gently tilts your pelvis, releasing your back and pulling in your tummy. It will help you if your tummy and back muscles are also weak.

You've now got your legs comfortably up in the air. Next turn them out. This means rotating the thigh outwards in the hip socket so that your heels come together and your knees face outwards. Tense your tummy muscles pressing your lower back into the floor. Slowly lower one leg keeping the other in its upright resting position. Lower the leg until you feel its weight being taken by your tummy muscles. That's far enough! Bring it back in to the resting position and lower the other leg. When your legs begin to feel tired bend them into your chest. Clasp your hands round your knees and pull your knees in towards you. This will release your legs and your back, as I described earlier. Try it with the breathing: breathe in then breathe out as you squeeze and pull in. Don't jerk at this movement.

As your legs and tummy become stronger you will be able to lower the legs further down but your back must never come off the floor! Remember you are starting from your point of strength and lowering down towards your point of weakness, so you should at all times have the control to pull up and out of this. Get the breathing to go with this. Always breathe in before you start and then breathe out as the leg goes down and in as it comes

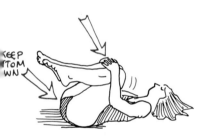

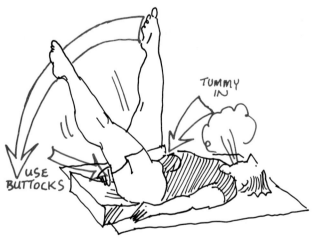

Single leg lowering

up. Once you have enough control to take the leg more than half-way down, then you can bring in the buttocks. The leg is (should be!) already turned out as you get past the half way down mark; squeeze in your buttocks, which will give you tremendous control from above and below so that instead of your leg wavering up and down it moves with strength at whatever speed you choose! Always bend your knees into your chest after each set of exercises.

DOUBLE LEG LOWERING (Chart Ex. 37)

This works on the same principle as the curl-down: starting from strength and going down to the weakest point. Bend your knees in and then lift into the air. Try stretching your feet (pointing your toes); it makes your legs look and work better. Turn your legs out, pull in your tummy and lower your legs until you feel

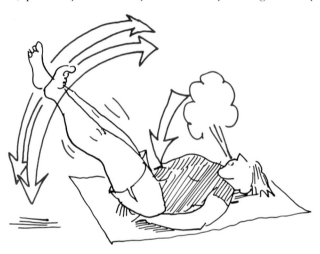

Double leg lowering, legs turned out (keep toes pointed)

the pull in your tummy muscles. Keep your back pressed into the floor throughout. This is much stronger because you have doubled the weight of your lever. Raise them up again, keeping the tummy pulled in. If you go too far you will feel it in your back (hip flexors again).

You may reach a stage where you feel you don't need the cushion but you're not quite ready to be flat on the floor. Try your hands under your bottom where your tail bone is. Just put one hand on top of the other and this will be enough to give your pelvis a gentle tilt. If you're not using your hands or a cushion, your back must stay on the floor all the time you are lowering and lifting your legs; your tummy should be pulled in, *not* quivering or bulging. Many people think an exercise is only doing them good if there is a lot of shaking and pain. The medicine doesn't *have* to taste bad to do you good, and there is a great difference between muscle glow and strain.

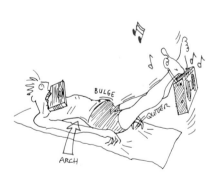

Wrong!

If you get your legs over halfway down, don't forget to bring in the buttocks. If you do get them all the way down, then your back will probably rise very slightly off the ground in the last stage. This is where you need to bring in the hip flexors at this floor-level point. That is why I think there is no point in getting your legs right down to the floor; you can do much more for your tummy muscles with them about halfway down – providing your tummy muscles are really pulled in!

SCISSORS (Chart Ex. 37)

This is just a stronger backwards and forwards version of the single leg lowering. It helps a lot here if your hamstrings are loosened up; if they are very tight, your leg won't come in towards you.

Bend your knees in, lift them into the air, then as you take one

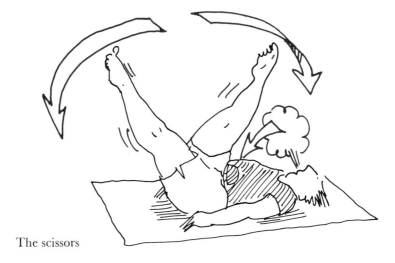

The scissors

leg forward bring the other leg back into you and then change them. This can be done quite fast so that the legs 'scissor' backwards and forwards. It is too quick to breathe in time to, so just breathe normally and don't hold your breath.

Whenever you start or finish an exercise with the legs, always bend them into your chest and take them up or down.

HEAD TO KNEE (Chart Ex. 38)

Try bending in one knee with your hands clasped round it and bringing your forehead to your knee. Release and then clasp your other knee and bring it into your forehead. Breathe out every time you bring the knee and forehead together. Keep the neck and shoulders relaxed. While you're working on the bent leg, your resting leg should be flat on the floor. To make the exercise harder you can raise the straight leg about four inches off the floor so that, as you change legs, the resting leg never touches the ground.

Head to knee – breathe out as you bring head to knee, other leg straight on floor

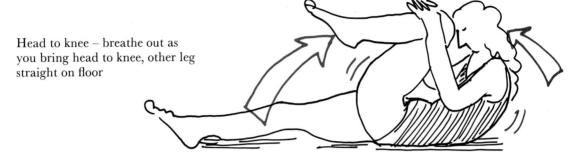

Head to knee (harder exercise) – keep resting leg 4 inches off floor

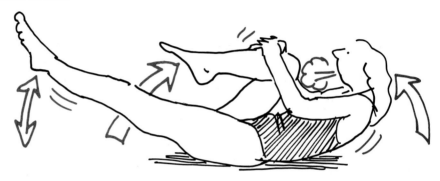

ELBOW TO KNEE (Chart Ex. 38)

Put your hands behind your head with your elbows out to the side. Bring your right elbow up to your left knee (working the obliques) breathing out, then go back to the floor breathing in. Next bring your left elbow up to your right knee and so on.

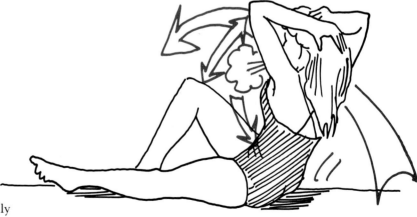

Elbow to knee, diagonally

There are all sorts of tummy muscle exercises. I have dealt with the simplest and safest, and tried to show you how to build up from there. All these exercises have been performed lying on your back, but you can work the tummy muscles sitting and standing too. Start with sitting – back to the hard chair or stool! The advantage of sitting is that you are supported.

SIDE BEND (Chart Ex. 13)

This works the tummy muscles at the side of the body and will help pull in your waist. Round your arms above your head keeping your shoulders down. The arms are being used to extend and add weight to the top half of the body so that you lengthen your lever. Now bend your trunk over to one side – if you are going to the right you should feel a pull up the left side of your body, from the hips up over the ribs. Make sure you are not leaning back, keep your tummy pulled in (not too much or you'll do a pelvic tilt!). Make small further movements to the side, trying to extend a bit more each time. Starting slowly pull up with the top elbow to help you get more lift – don't jerk. Try to release into it. If your bottom rises up off the stool on one side, place your legs further apart to give you a more solid base. Finally come up to the centre, bring your arms down and circle your shoulders to release them. If you felt tension building up in your neck, don't force your head

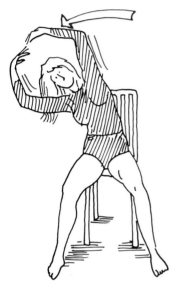

Side bend – a good waist exercise

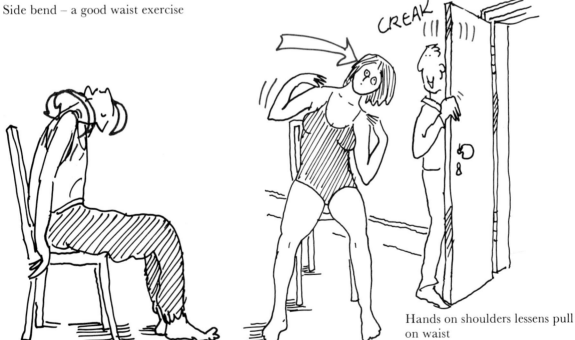

Hands on shoulders lessens pull on waist

Circle your shoulders, head forwards

back and shorten up those muscles even more. Let your head go forward a little. Raise your arm again and repeat to the other

69

side. If you are very weak or have a rigid neck and shoulders, you can either rest your hands on your head or on your shoulders. Resting them on your shoulders also makes it less of a pull on the waist. Less leverage!

WAIST TWISTS (Chart Ex. 14)

This is very important not only for the tummy muscles but also for the mobility of the spine. Rest your hands on your chest with your elbows relaxed at your side. Lengthen the back of your neck and turn your head round over your right shoulder. Don't let the head tilt. Now turn your back around as if you were pivoting on a steel rod through the centre of your body. This pivoting feeling should stop you leaning back. Pulling in your tummy muscles and lifting your ribs will also help to make your 'waist' muscles work harder. Use your back shoulder to help lever you round, so when you are turning to the right pull back (not up – keep the shoulder down) with your right shoulder. Try to see the wall behind you by looking out of the corner of your eyes (without squinting!). This will also exercise your eyes, remembering that they too have muscles. Aim to get your hips square forwards and your shoulder at a right angle to them square to the wall to your right, when you are turning in that direction, and to the left when you reverse the movement.

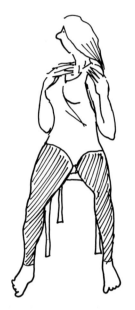

Waist twist (tummy muscles pulled in)

DIAGONAL BEND (Chart Ex. 15)

When you bend and twist your spine at the same time it puts an extra strain on it. This is perfectly safely held by a normal spine, but if there is a weakness in your lower back this should either be left out or attempted with caution.

Lift your arms and round them over your head as in side bends. Turn the top half of your body to the right. Pull in your left-side tummy muscles and take your left elbow over towards and beyond your left knee. Imagine that there is a bar at your waist which you have to lift up and over. If your elbow reaches or goes down beyond your knee, you have lost the pull-in in the left tummy muscles so start again to get the lift. Once you have the correct pull-in, you will feel a stretch up the right side of your back. The more you pull in on the left, the more you will be able to stretch out on your right. Try not to swing your body up and down in this position but keep to a smaller range of further movements, all the time trying to extend the body further by pulling in the side tummy muscles, pulling up with the top elbow and reaching forwards with the arms. It's a lot to remember; try practising in front of a mirror.

When you want to stop, come up in the twisted position, turn to the front, lower your arms and circle your shoulders to release. Then lift your arms up again and drop your shoulders, turn to

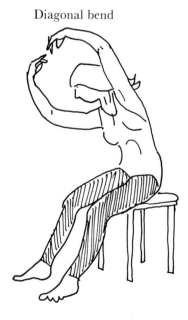

Diagonal bend

70

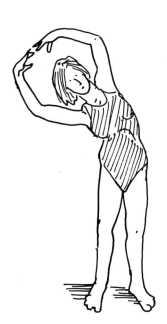

Side bend standing up

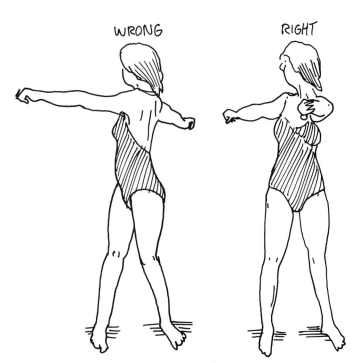

WRONG   RIGHT

Keep hips central when doing the waist twist

your left, pull in on the right and reach forward beyond the right knee pulling up with the left elbow. Come up in the twisted position arms down, circle the shoulders and relax.

Both the side bend and the twist can be performed standing up. This is fine if your base is still firm. But the side bend is only effective if the hips are kept central and not allowed to sway out to the side. If the hips and knees swing with the twist, this can cause problems with the spine as well as making the exercise ineffective, so remember to centre your pelvis and pull up above the knees when performing these two movements standing. Also make sure that the weight is evenly distributed through the feet as in correct standing.

THE 'RUDE' BIT

I have called this section the 'rude' bit to encompass a whole area of the anatomy some people seem reticent to talk about. Although this book is very definitely *not* for women only, this section is perhaps more relevant to their particular anatomical arrangement. The muscles I am now dealing with in particular are the perineum muscles or the pelvic floor. We all have pelvic floors and we all have anal passages and urethras, but then we get to the big difference between men and women.

First let's look at what a pelvic floor is. Basically, it is the sling of muscles in layers which hold up the lower part of the abdominal contents in the pelvic basin. This means that these muscles must be in a permanent state of contraction. These are mainly involuntary muscles. But there are also voluntary muscles which can be pulled up.

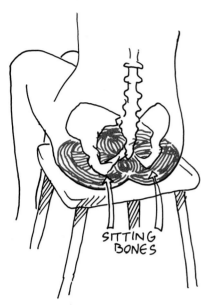

Showing the pelvic floor and sitting bones

The pelvic floor is penetrated by the orifices which in turn are surrounded by sphincter muscles. These loop around the anus at the back and the urethra and vagina in front, forming a sort of figure of eight. The anus is the strongest sphincter muscle, but the loop around the urethra and vagina is the 'master' muscle. You cannot contract one loop without the other, so all the orifices will squeeze together. The best exercise, therefore, to discover these muscles is to stop when you are halfway through passing water, rather like turning off a tap! Once you have found these muscles, use them frequently, squeezing then releasing them.

What happens, though, if you can't 'turn off the tap'? Sometimes the pelvic floor weakens in quite young women, but normally it is in the later years through neglect and childbearing that problems begin to manifest themselves. A healthy pelvic floor should be taut, with the muscles held firmly from the pubic bone in front to the coccyx (tail bone) at the back. These hold the bladder, uterus (womb) and anus at an angle to their relevant passages (urethra and vagina). When the muscles weaken from the pressures that are put on them – remember the abdominal plus pressure then add coughing, sneezing, jumping, excreting, etc. – the pelvic floor sags and this changes the angle of the bladder, uterus and anus tilting them up so that they become prone to prolapse. The weakened sphincter muscles also mean loss of control so that incontinence can become a real and unpleasant problem.

Many doctors tell women that this is the norm at their age and recommend surgery as the remedy but there is almost always an alternative, the pelvic floor exercise, if you catch this early enough. And yet most pople have never heard of their pelvic floors or been given any indication that they could and should be exercised. One doctor in America has done a great deal of research into the action of the pelvic floor. He is Dr Arnold Kegal and pelvic floor contractions have even become known as the Kegal exercise. It is normally possible to tighten up these muscles through exercise when they have become slack and to bring them back to their correct position. This in turn will readjust the position of the bladder, uterus or anus so that they return to their normal angle.

It is never too late or too early to start exercising the pelvic floor. I do my pelvic floor contractions while waiting at the supermarket check-out, or sitting in a traffic jam. But they are probably best learnt in a lying position so that you don't have the weight of the abdominal organs or the pull of gravity to work against.

PELVIC FLOOR PULL-UPS (With Chart Ex. 29, or any time)

Lie on your back with your knees bent and your feet flat on the floor. Draw up the pelvic floor and grip with the sphincter muscles until you feel the inside passages tighten up. If you put your hands over your pubic bone it helps you to 'think' into tightening all the way up the vagina. Hold for two or three seconds and then

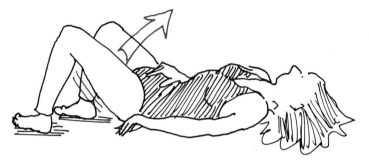

The pelvic floor pull-up

release. You can do a succession of quick contractions and then rest – but always end up with a contraction. It's quite a good idea to combine this exercise with a pelvic tilt so that you get the feeling of *everything* pulling in. I would recommend fifty pelvic floor contractions a day to get those muscles really strong again (remembering that little and often is most effective rather than trying to do them all at once). Try to incorporate them in your daily life as I have suggested.

Pelvic floor lifts will give you a bit more to think about, and are the most strengthening pelvic floor exercises. You can start lying down and then progress to anywhere, any time, any position, once you've got the hang of it. Try to control the squeeze of your vagina, starting at the bottom as if you were going up in a lift. Slowly take yourself up floor by floor. Don't lose control when you've reached the top, try to hold for a slow count of four then let yourself down slowly, stage by stage.

If you do have problems with prolapse (a looseness in the pelvic floor) do try and exercise it back even though it may take more time and effort. It is well worth it. If you haven't yet experienced any problem in that area, remember you're dealing with a muscle like any other and without exercise it will eventually lose its elasticity. Degeneration is slow, so don't rest on your laurels because you've not had any problems yet. Anyway, I think these exercises are fun, so enjoy them!

6 Thigh High to Knees

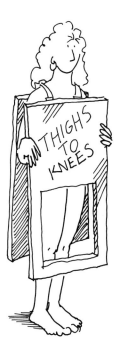

I suppose we would all like long, lean thighs but first their shape is determined by the length of their bone, the femur. Some people have long legs, some long bodies and that's to do with your body type, so you can't change that. Also the basic shape of the thigh muscles depends on whether you are a mesomorph endomorph or ectomorph. If your thighs are muscularly well developed, they are never going to pare down to skinny sticks. Thighs are also one of the first places women put weight on and in many women this fact manifests itself by dimpley bumps we call cellulite. Weak thighs tend to bulge out round the side – the French call them 'culotte de cheval' (jodhpurs) – and are more prone to collecting fat.

Okay, you can't change the basic structure of your thighs, but you can certainly improve on the shape by stretching them fully, and you will get a lot more leg power by using them properly in everyday life.

Once again the weight problem must be tackled with diet, as well as exercise, including the control of cellulite. One of the ladies appearing with me on my television programme had previously allowed herself to get enormous – 'square' as she described it. After following the weight watchers régime, one of the first things she lost was inches off each thigh.

If you want to judge how much weight you have put on, keep an eye on your thighs. I don't possess any bathroom scales but I always know when I've put on weight by the tightness of my jeans. If the jeans are feeling a bit tight, sure enough there is the extra couple of pounds if I weigh myself. And that's the time to lose them. It's easy come, easy go. If you leave the pounds and let them establish themselves and then put on a few more and a few more, it's going to take a lot more effort to get off the stones.

I'm not totally advocating that American saying 'you can never be too thin or too rich'. I don't know about the being too rich part, but certainly you can be too thin. Thinness can become obsessive and this is not healthy. It is often not attractive, either. In its extreme it is the anorexic, unable to eat, revolted by food and by him- or herself, with a body weight of a few stone. This kind of thinness can lead to death. Others are less extreme in their dieting, but still try to diet below their natural weight and end up looking scraggy. This is particularly true of older women. I am *not* saying that you can get away with middle-age spread and should let your body go because 'that's what happens to people of my age'. I am just trying to get you to see weight and body shape realistically. Weight has a lot to do with the state of your mind. Most people under pressure turn to food; fat people are not all the jolly souls we imagine, although outwardly that's the way they may appear. That is why I am writing a book about your emotional states and how you cope with them. If you get your head right, the dieting part will be much easier. Mind and body are one, whether you like it or not. Taking care of one will take care of the other. So let's get on with a bit of exercise to get things moving.

Thighs are made up of front, back, inside and outside sets of muscles. The main front and back groups of muscles work together as do the ones at either side.

The muscle group at the front of the thigh is the quadriceps (*rectus femoris*, *vastus lateralis* and *vastus medialis*). The longest muscle in the body, the *sartorius*, also passes diagonally over the front of the thigh. At the back of the thigh are the hamstrings (*biceps femoris, semimembranosus* and *semitendinosus*). On the inside of the thigh are the *adductor* muscles and the *gracilis* muscle and the outside thigh is made up of the gluteal muscles, abductors, which come down from the buttocks. That's why, when you let your buttocks get weak (as happens when you spend too much time sitting), the result is a bulge round to the side of the thighs – the jodhpurs look.

The thigh muscles were made to be strong. The legs support the trunk and they get us around. I have divided the legs into their two natural halves because I think each half deserves separate attention. This chapter is called 'Thigh high to knees' because it is the muscles of the thigh which move the knee joint. The hamstrings flex the knee (take the lower leg back) whilst the quadriceps extend the knee joint (bring the lower leg forward). The knee joint is a hinge joint and if it wasn't for the knee cap or patella it would hinge in both directions. The knee is held in place by strong ligaments but has very little muscle surrounding it. This makes it a vulnerable joint and is why it is so prone to injury. In addition, it is a main weight-bearing joint and can be pushed into some pretty odd positions, particularly when playing sports. The quadriceps surround only the top part of the knee (fat knees = weak quadriceps), so when the knee is injured or weakened you will be given exercises to strengthen the quadriceps. To shock-absorb the jolts and jars on the knee, the joint contains numerous pads of fat and bursae. Bursae are small sacs of viscous fluid rather like water cushions. When these become inflamed it is called housemaid's knee. Prolonged kneeling can cause this kind of injury, so try not to kneel for too long, and always use a pad!

The knee, like other joints, also contains synovial fluid which lubricates the joints. Occasionally the synovial membrane becomes inflamed. This is synovitis which is more commonly known as tennis elbow because the inflammation is caused by jarring the joint. You can also get tennis elbow in the knee! Another knee problem, often found in sportsmen, is a toughening of the cartilage on the inside of the kneecap. Basically, it is caused by an imbalance in the quadricep muscles through always working with the knees bent. Squatting in weightlifting, hurdling, rowing and bounding along all require strong quadriceps, but they all use

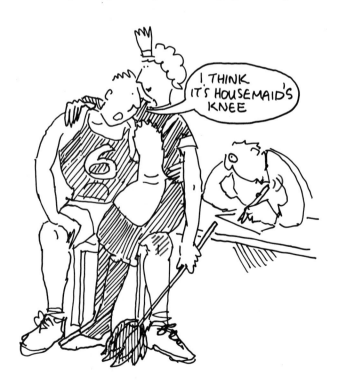

bent knees. If the knee is not straightened enough, the *vastus medialis* becomes weak and puts the kneecap out of alignment; this then grates away against the thigh bone (femur) and causes a lot of pain.

Don't try to diagnose your own knee injury. The knee is a delicate structure and needs medical diagnosis and treatment. If your knees are just rather weak or fat, this is how to work them.

SITTING WITH LEGS STRAIGHT FORWARD (Chart Ex. 55)

First take the weight off your knees by sitting on the floor. Stretch your legs straight out in front of you. If you feel a strong pull at the back of your legs, then your hamstrings desperately need stretching – most people feel some kind of pull at first. You can sit against a wall to support your back. Now flex your feet (pull your toes up towards you) until your heels come off the floor. It is the quadriceps shortening and tightening which are pulling up around your knee. At the same time you will feel a pull (strong pull) right down the back of your legs – the muscles are stretching! If your heels are not coming off the ground, it could be because the muscles at the back are too tight (see exercises to stretch the hamstring) or that the *vastus medialis* is weak. Either way, keep going with this exercise.

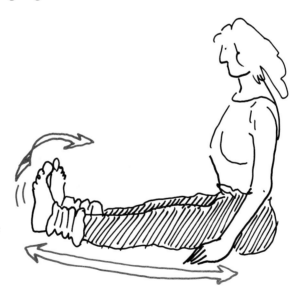

Quadriceps exercise to strengthen knees: first stage

When you feel the quadriceps have strengthened sufficiently, you can try something a bit stronger (if you are under treatment, let the doctor or physiotherapist decide when you are ready for this). Sit on the edge of a bed or chair with your leg straight out in front of you. Add weight at the ankle and then raise the leg up and down so you can feel it in the front of the thigh. Weight can be added by filling two bags with sugar or beans and attaching them with string. This way you can increase or decrease the weight by taking out or adding more beans. (A personal note: if you use sugar I would throw it away afterwards – I don't keep any in the house! – use honey or molasses for sweetening where necessary.)

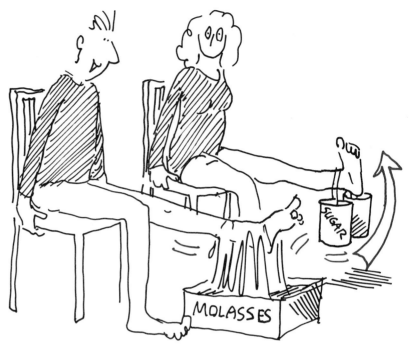

Quadriceps exercise to strengthen knees: second stage

Once you've got your knees back to full strength you can try other exercises for strengthening the quadriceps. But these involve putting weight in the knees, so any pain in the joints should be taken seriously and these exercises should then be left out.

You can get your thighs going sitting down. This sounds rather lazy but it can be very hard work. Back to your hard chair or stool again. If your thighs are pretty weak, sit right back so that most of the thigh is supported by the seat. As your thigh gets stronger and you need less support for your leg then you can start to move forward a bit until you are sitting on the edge of your seat. Your tummy muscles will also need to be strong enough to hold you in this position.

SITTING LEG KICKS (Chart Ex. 16)

Tilt your hips back by pulling in your tummy muscles (with your back released you should not feel any pull there. If you do feel anything in your back, you are not holding the weight of your leg in your tummy muscles so come up and start again). Put your hands on your hips with your finger tips firmly on your tummy, if the muscles begin to weaken you will feel them with your sensitive fingers! Now lift your leg up and turn it out with your foot flexed. The leg should come about halfway up from the floor.

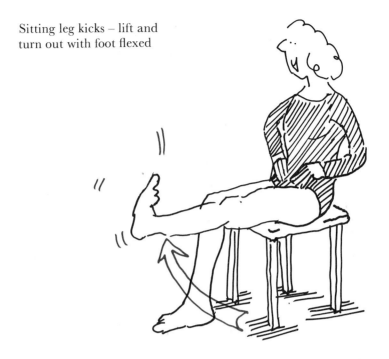

Sitting leg kicks – lift and turn out with foot flexed

Turning it out will help control it from underneath. Don't bend your knee in too far but enough to be able to kick the leg forcefully. If there is any discomfort in the knee joint don't go on kicking the leg, just bend it and straighten it giving you the same muscle work without jarring the weakened joint.

Normal knees carry on kicking. Small bend, strong kick. Don't worry if you see your thighs wobbling! Even tiny, thin, firm thighs will quiver with the force of the kick so don't hold back in horror at all that wobbling flesh; get some life into it. I like to start off with some slow kicks and then (if there is no pain in the joint) speed them up to get the circulation really going. This can be surprisingly exhausting! Be careful that your shoulders don't come up unnoticed as you concentrate on your leg.

When you have worked one leg, come back to your upright position, take a deep breath and then tilt your hips and lift your other leg making sure you turn it out and flex the foot. Watch out for the foot of the 'resting' leg too. Make sure it is resting and not lifted up off the floor.

This is a very good thigh exercise as it can be done comfortably sitting down and the thigh is strengthened and straightened.

The next two thigh exercises are much stronger and I have

followed both with quadriceps stretches. There must always be a balance in muscles between the stretch and the strength. It is no good having super strong solid muscles with no stretch. Apart from anything else they become a hideous shape, all short and bulky. If a muscle is not stretched out to its full length again after it has been contracted, this is what happens. On the other hand if you only concentrate on stretching muscles, they will become weak. When you see someone who is very loose and whose legs seem to go in any direction you must remember that this also indicates a looseness of the ligaments which hold the joint in place. If the ligaments are too loose, the joint can slip round and the bones will eventually grate away wearing down the cartilage and cause inflammation and degeneration of the joint. It is therefore particularly important that the muscles surrounding the joint should be kept strong enough to help hold everything in place.

STANDING QUADRICEPS STRENGTHENER (Chart Ex. 27)

To strengthen the quadriceps standing up, use the back of a chair or a table top for balance; stand with the inside of your feet

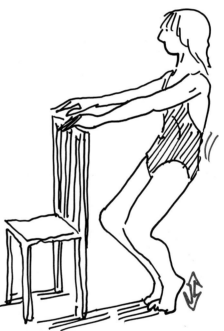

Standing quadriceps strengthener, using chair for balance

together, then rise up onto the balls of your feet. (The chair or table will help to keep you balanced if you rest your fingers on a solid surface!) Bend your knees letting them drop apart and tilt your pelvis so that your tummy is scooped out and your back curled under. Now push forwards and down with your knees until you feel the weight of your body in your thighs. This exercise is very good preparation for skiing. Come up when you feel that the muscles have had enough – a good glow at least.

STANDING QUADRICEPS STRETCH (Chart Ex. 2)

To stretch the thighs after this contraction, straighten right up and stand on one leg. Bend the other leg up behind you, catch hold of the foot or ankle and gently pull the foot in towards you.

Keep the supporting leg (the one you are standing on!) straight. Don't arch your back to get your bent leg into you, but push forward with your hips (pelvic tilt) even if your knee doesn't come in quite so far. Don't pull too hard on your leg, this is supposed to be a release for the quadriceps not pulling the knee out of its socket! When you have stretched the front of your thigh change over and bend the other leg up in the same way. At first you will need to rest one hand on the chair or table for support but eventually you should be able to stand on one leg and pull the other one up behind without holding on.

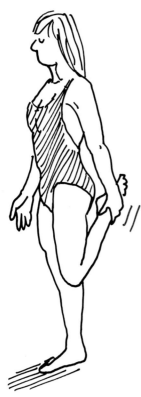

Standing quadriceps stretch

HINGING (Chart Ex. 51)

This is done kneeling on the floor. If the floor is very hard, put a small cushion or lightly folded towel under your knees first. The knees should be slightly apart (about hip width). Start kneeling upright, with your arms stretched out in front of you. Now grip with your buttocks really tightly and pull in your tummy so that

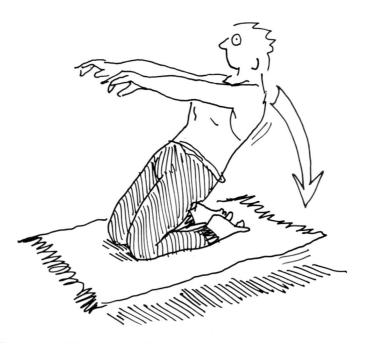

Hinging – holding weight of body in quadriceps

your centre is very strong. (Imagine there is a board down your back so that you can't bend!) Keeping your body absolutely straight, slowly lean backwards holding the weight of your body in your quadriceps. You will soon feel this if you are doing it properly. Don't go too far or overdo this one at first as it is very strong and you could end up with stiff thighs (I did once)! Come up slowly with your body still holding its straight position. I usually count slowly to four going down and four coming up. I think that four sets of this exercise is enough at any one time unless you particularly need to build up this area. But remember this is not an exercise for weak knees.

HINGE RELEASE (Chart Ex. 52)

To stretch the thighs after the hinge, take your right leg forward with knee bent. Don't let the knee push forwards beyond the

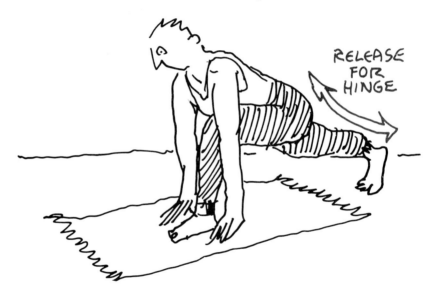

Hinge release – stage 1: rest body over front thigh

heel. Now hinge your left leg back as far as it will go, with the ball of the foot resting on the floor. Rest your body over the front thigh without letting the knee push forwards, which would put it in a vulnerable position. Move the back leg further away from you to increase the stretch, bend in the leg that is behind you (you started with the left leg behind), catch hold of your left foot or ankle with your right hand and gently draw it in towards you. Make sure that this back knee is also on your towel or cushion and not on a hard floor (carpet will do).

Release the foot when you feel you have stretched enough, then change legs. Left leg bent in front of you, knee over heel; right leg lunged back behind you. If this stretch is enough, there is no need to go on to the next stage. For the really strong stretch

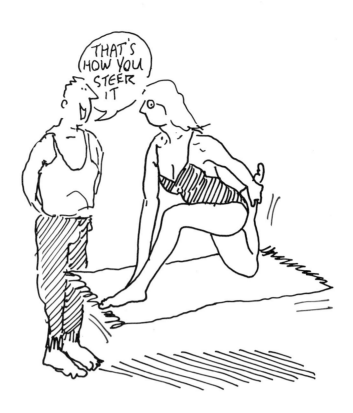

Hinge release – stage 2:
move back leg further back
and draw in foot with
opposite hand

bend in your right foot and catch hold of it with your left hand;
draw it in as far as you can, then release. The following two exercises will help to pull in those bulging bits at the side of the thighs
and strengthen the muscles around the hips, helping to keep the
joint firm and in place. Combined with the other buttock exercises they will help to pull in your bottom and the backs of your
thighs and tighten them up. The second squeeze also gets into the
fatty part of the hips which will increase the circulation in this
area as you get the muscles working.

THIGH EXERCISE 1: LYING DOWN (Chart Ex. 39)

Lie on your side, stretching your underneath arm away from your
underneath leg so that your body is straight. Rest your top arm
on the floor at chest level to balance you. Keep your tummy
muscles working, even though you are lying on the floor, to
maintain this straight position. If you find it more comfortable,
you can prop your head up by bending in your underneath arm,
but don't take your body off the ground by coming right up on to
your elbow. Lift the top leg up to the side and rotate it inwards.
First try turning the thigh inwards and outwards in the hip socket
a few times, then you'll get the feel of it. With the leg turned inwards flex the foot and swing the leg upwards. Don't let it come all

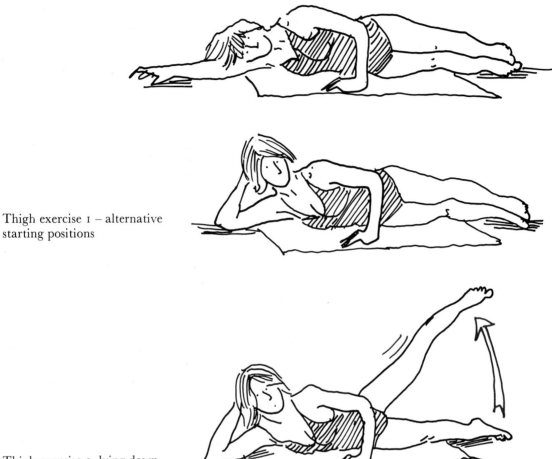

Thigh exercise 1 – alternative
starting positions

Thigh exercise 1, lying down –
lift top leg and rotate inwards

the way down; just enough to release before you take it up again.
Now it is very important that the leg is going up to the side; you
should be able to feel this up the outside thigh and squeezing into
the hip. The mistake that most people make at first is that they
allow their body to roll slightly back and their leg to lift slightly
forwards. This immediately takes the work from the side of the
thigh to the front of the thigh (this is cheating!). It is an ineffectual
exercise for the front of the thigh and does nothing for the weak
muscles at the side of the thigh, which you are trying to get to.

Looking in a mirror can help you to see if you are going wrong.
Then try to 'feel' which muscles you are using. Another reason
many people find this hard is bony hips! If your underneath hip is
sticking into the floor, you naturally want to roll back a bit to get
off it. To alleviate this or just to give you a more solid base to
start off with, bend in your underneath leg. Before you do this
take your leg down so that you can start from the beginning – body

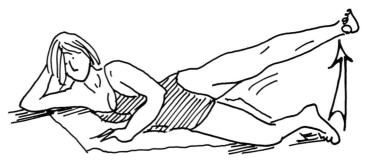

Thigh exercise 1, lying down – with underneath leg bent for more solid base

and legs straight out along the floor, top arm at chest level for balance, tummy pulled in to keep the centre strong. Bend the underneath leg so that the knee half sticks out beyond the top leg and the foot end sticks out behind in equal parts. If you get the leg out more in front, you will tend to 'banana' and roll the body back so that the top leg would come forwards. If the bottom leg is bent too far behind, it will make you arch back so that the top leg would go too far behind. Press the toes of your underneath foot into the floor so that the heel lifts; your leg is now 'on the walk'. Next try lifting your top leg again and turning it in. Flex the foot, pull up above the knee to keep the leg straight and swing the leg up and halfway down. Keeping the leg straight is very important for working the thigh. If the knee is bent, you are trying to do all the work with your foot and calf. If you get cramp in your foot or calf with the foot flexed, just relax or stretch it. You are again trying to bypass the thigh muscles and are trying to put all the work into the foot and calf muscles instead. When you lower your leg to rest it, bend both knees up into you to release your muscles.

If your muscles are not very strong, roll over onto your other side so that you can work your other leg in the same way, then turn over onto the first side for the second exercise. However, once you have strengthened up a bit you should be able to follow the first exercise with the second, after a quick release, without having to change legs. So you do two exercises on one leg, then turn over and do two on the other leg in the same way.

THIGH EXERCISE 2: LYING DOWN (Chart Ex. 40)

Lie on your side and lift your top leg halfway up from the floor, swing it back and at the same time roll the top half of your body

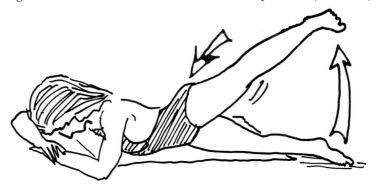

Thigh exercise 2, lying down – relaxed top of body, hip forward, leg back, foot flexed – rotate leg outwards

forwards so that you are resting on your chest with your elbows on either side and your head on your hands. This should be a relaxed position for the top part of your body. The important thing is that your hip should be forward and your leg should be back with the foot flexed. If you can rotate the leg outwards without moving the position of your hip, so much the better, but don't worry too much about this. At first concentrate on the basic position.

Now push your leg up and back squeezing up and into the back of the hip; release halfway down and push up again. This should feel much stronger and more concentrated than the first exercise. This is because you are working into a little-used muscle which is one of the reasons fat easily collects there. Again, be careful that you don't allow your knee to bend; you must work from your thigh with the calf and foot following passively.

To finish, release in the same way as the first exercise by bringing your leg down and bending both knees in. This will stop you holding any tension in your muscles. Don't forget to work both sides.

Both those exercises can be done standing up. It is easier to cheat standing up and it is harder to do them correctly, so do make sure you know the 'feel' of the muscle work before you try this.

THIGH EXERCISE 1: STANDING (Chart Ex. 24)

Use the back of a chair or a table to rest your fingers on for balance. Do not cling on or rest your weight into whatever you are using, it's not a prop!

With your left hand resting on the table lift your right hip and heel. This contracts the hip. Now lift your leg to the side keeping it turned inwards with the foot flexed. It should not come up too far before you feel the squeeze in your hip. If you rest your hand on your hip, you should be able to feel it contract. Make sure your tummy is pulling in so that you are not arching your back and so that you are not leaning towards the table and away from your working leg (the one you are lifting). If you lean away from the working leg, you will have nothing to squeeze into, so it is important to keep the supporting leg straight and the body pulled up. Pulling up your body will also help to take some of the weight out of your supporting leg. Be careful not to pull up your shoulders, though. Lift the working leg up into the hip as far as you can and then release it halfway down. Try this at different speeds. A few slow ones for control and to work deep into the muscle and quicker ones for the surface muscles and to get everything going. Try taking your hand away from your chair or table half way through this exercise just to make sure you are not leaning towards it and can balance for a short while without any support. To release your leg, bend the knee up and clasp it into you.

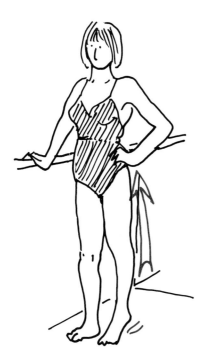

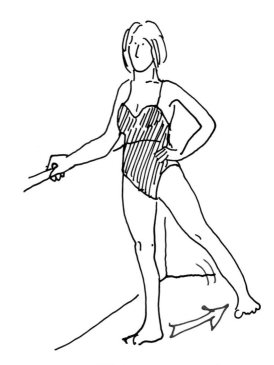

Thigh exercise 1, standing –
starting position: lift outside
hip and heel (hip contraction)

Thigh exercise 1, standing –
lift leg to side, rotate inwards,
foot flexed

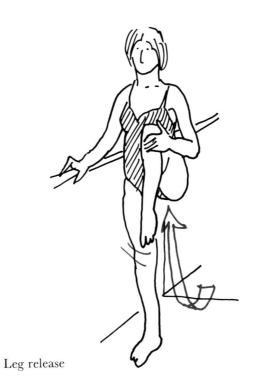

Leg release

Turn around and work the other leg in the same way. It is doubly important to pull up and out of the supporting leg this time as this is now the leg you have just worked so you may feel more in this leg than the actual working leg. This will pass as the thighs strengthen. Don't forget to lift the hip and heel before lifting your leg and to flex your foot and turn the leg inwards.

A quick word of warning here on the 'sickle' position of your foot. A 'sickle' foot is a foot that turns inwards. It is not attractive looking and it also weakens the outside ankle. So when I ask you to turn your leg in with a flexed foot, do be careful to keep the foot straight and not to turn it in or 'sickle' it. This applies to all the leg exercises, so keep an eye on your feet!

THIGH EXERCISE 2: STANDING (Chart Ex. 25)

This exercise is best done facing your chair or table. Rest your finger tips on the back of the chair or table and make sure that your hips face it squarely. Lift your right hip and heel and take your leg diagonally back. Pull in your tummy to centre your pelvis so that your back doesn't arch, and be careful not to let your hips open out – in other words, keep both hips squarely forwards!

It's important that you keep your body position as firm as it was when it was supported by the floor in both these exercises.

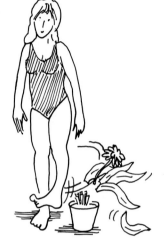

'Sickle' position of foot

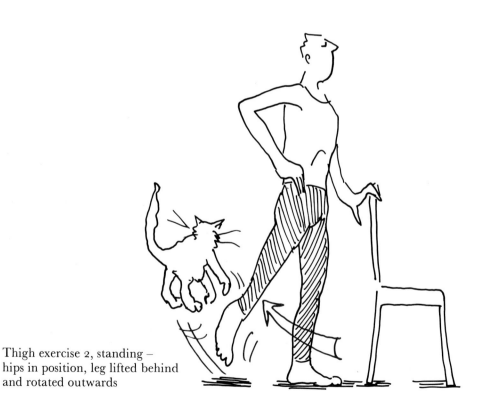

Thigh exercise 2, standing –
hips in position, leg lifted behind
and rotated outwards

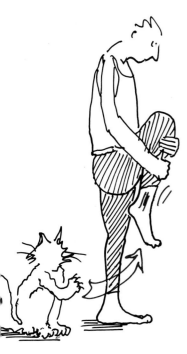

Thigh release

You can cheat (yourself!) if you allow your body to lean away from the leg you are lifting since you then have nothing to push against. One of the reasons that the standing positions are so much harder is that you have to use many more muscles to keep the body position.

Now your leg is diagonally back behind you, see if you can turn it out from the hip. You don't have to worry about the foot in outward rotations; it will only 'sickle' when you turn the leg in (or sometimes when the leg is straight, but I will deal with that later). Keep the hips in position and then lift your leg up behind, as far as you can, release halfway down and push up again. Keep going, feeling the squeeze up in the back of the hip as you push up. When you've done enough (don't overdo it at first otherwise you won't have the strength to stand on that leg while you work the other one) bend your knee in and then change legs.

Remember to pull in your tummy and lift the hip and heel before you take the leg back, so that your starting position is strong. Turn the leg out, flex the foot and keep lifting up and diagonally back with a straight leg. Vary the speed of the lifts.

Even after lifting your knee, when you have finished you may still feel very tight at the top of your hips and in the lower back where you have worked the muscles. Try some flat back release.

THE FLAT BACK RELEASE (Chart Ex. 26)

Stretch your arms out away from the chair back or table so that your back flattens and your legs come straight down from your hips with the feet slightly apart. Make sure the legs are not too far forward or too far back but directly under your hips. Try to relax your back in this position so that it is flat like a table top,

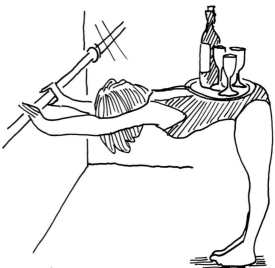

The flat back release – legs directly under hips, bounce gently on arms

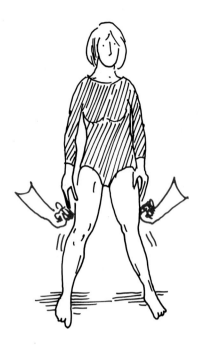

not all rounded up or sunk down in the middle with your tummy hanging out. This is a good stretch for your arms and shoulders too and you can *gently* bounce on the arms, if you don't feel too much pull in the still position. You may feel this stretching your lower back if it is stiff, or the backs of your thighs (hamstrings) if they are very tight. Try doing a pelvic tilt in this position as this will release your back further and give your tummy muscles an extra pull in (and because I never miss an opportunity to do a pelvic tilt!). Keep the top part of your back flat and pull in your tummy muscles. The pelvis will only tilt very slightly in this position, but it is enough! You will have quite forgotten all your leg work when you come up from this position.

INSIDE THIGH SQUEEZE (Chart Ex. 28)

While you are still standing just try this exercise (inside thigh squeeze). Feet slightly apart, pelvis centred (pull in your tummy), press inwards with the inside thighs so that you can feel them grip. Release and grip again, and so on. You will feel your buttocks squeeze in sympathy with each grip, just as you felt the inside thigh work each time you did your buttock exercise on the stool.

Inside thigh squeeze – squeezing buttocks and pulling in tummy muscles, press inwards with inside thighs

LYING LEG KICKS (Chart Ex. 33)

This involves getting into the same position as we used for the tummy exercises. Flat on your back on the floor, bending in your knees, legs together straight up in the air and turned out for the

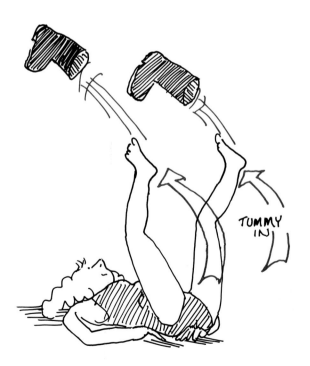

Lying leg kicks – legs straight up and turned out, kick out forcefully

resting position. Don't forget to place your hands under your bottom or a cushion, if necessary. Really stretch your feet out, point your toes. Part the legs halfway, bend them slightly and then kick them out forcefully. Keep up a good pace, watching out for the knees. Really try to stretch the feet out and away from you each time so that the leg elongates. Don't forget to keep your tummy muscles pulled in.

THE 'FROG' (Chart Ex. 34)

When your legs feel good and warm (tired!) bring them together and bend them into your chest, clasp your hands round the outside of each knee and draw them apart keeping your toes together. Now draw your knees back in towards your arm pits without your bottom coming off the floor. After you have squeezed the knees in, bring them down (still apart) and rest your toes on the floor as close as you can. Keep the heels lifted off the ground. Gently bounce your knees apart. You can rest your hands on the inside of your thighs to help to push them apart. This will help to open up the inside thigh and the hip socket. Draw your knees back in again and bring the legs up to the resting position.

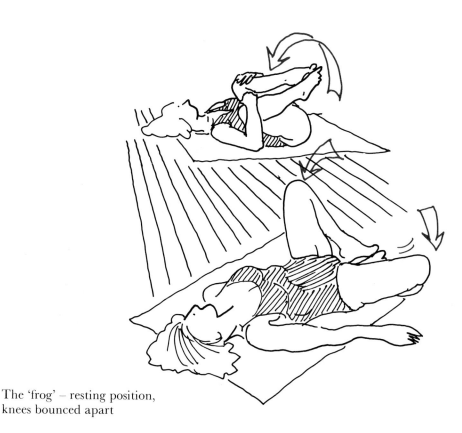

The 'frog' – resting position, knees bounced apart

LEGS APART IN THE AIR (Chart Ex. 35)

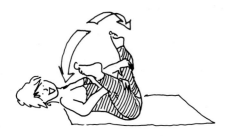

Legs apart in the air – working inside thighs

This works the inside thigh. Stretch your legs and feet and turn them out so the heels come together; now drop your legs apart, making sure that they don't drop forwards. If they are going forwards it is probably because the hamstrings are too tight and are pulling them away from you, or you are too weak to hold them up for long. To help prevent this, use your hands or a cushion under your pelvis as you did for the tummy muscle exercises, or rest your hands on the inside of your thighs just above the knees. With your hands in this position you can also help to encourage the thighs further apart. You can either hold this position or bounce the legs, but make sure they are really stretched out – they will work better and look much more elegant! Having given them a good stretch bring your legs together, bend them into your chest and rest them by squeezing them into your chest as you did between tummy muscle exercises.

To stretch and strengthen the inside thighs bring your legs up again, turn them out and drop them apart. Now bring them back together and then drop them out, and in and out and so on. Try this slowly and fast or try dropping them loosely out and then squeezing them slowly in (this is the strengthening part). If you have a friend handy they can help you strengthen your thighs by

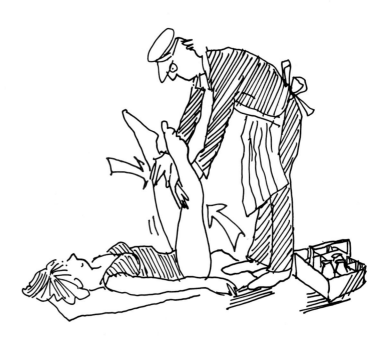

Legs apart in the air – strengthening thighs with the help of a 'friend'

placing their hands on the inside of your calves while your legs are apart. Now you have to squeeze your thighs together while your friend resists with his or her hands. Don't strain and hold your breath!

So far, we have mainly dealt with strengthening the thighs but it is equally important to keep them stretched, not only to keep the muscles fully lengthened but also to stimulate their stretch reflex. The stretch reflex is what stimulates the springiness or tone of the muscle. The more you stretch a muscle, the more it will spring back into place. Therefore if you want to stretch and open out a tight muscle you must be careful *how* you stretch it. On the other hand, if you are worried about your muscles becoming stretched like old elastic, this won't happen while you are using them. Muscles only weaken and atrophy when they are not used.

To stretch a tight muscle, it is important to hold the stretch and not just bounce at it all the time. So to stretch a muscle you must open it out gently, firmly and slowly especially at first. Once the muscle has started to stretch, bouncing (especially with music which makes it more rythmical and fun) is a good way to warm up and increase the stretch. Bouncing on tight muscle only jerks at it, not allowing it time to sustain its stretch, sometimes over-stimulating the stretch reflex and occasionally damaging it by straining or tearing it. So go easy at first. Strengthening, on the other hand, is better done with a movement than by holding a contraction. In isometric exercises you contract the muscle statically but it has been found that holding this kind of contraction for too long builds up negative tension and may leave the muscle in spasm. I find, therefore, that as a general rule stretches are better performed slowly and strengthened with a movement.

The next three exercises are mainly working on stretching the thighs, but as they are performed in a sitting position on the floor they require a certain amount of work in the back. Some people find the back work the hardest, so I would like to explain it before we begin the stretches.

From the age when we first sit behind a school desk and bend over our work, the back muscles are being held in a rounded

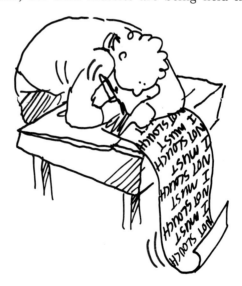

position. Even if you were encouraged to sit up straight it would be a tremendous strain on the muscles to maintain this for such a long period of time and inevitably after a while the body begins to slump forward. This is why typist chairs are designed to support the back and made adjustable for different body lengths. The

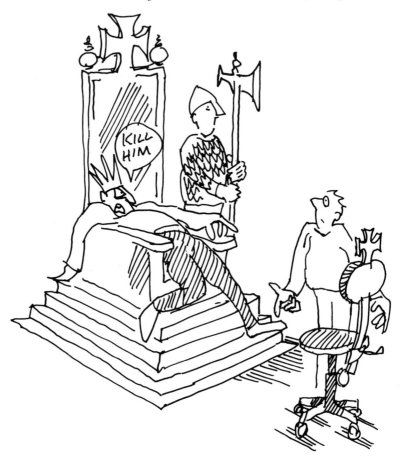

back of the chair should correspond with the muscles which hold the body upright. These are the *erector spinae* and a great girdle of muscle called the *latisimus dorsai*. Unfortunately most chairs are designed for their looks or for economy but with little thought for the needs of the body. I once met a writer who was coming close to a deadline, with a great deal of work still to be done. He spent long hours cramped non-stop over his desk with the result that his back became extremely painful and even his knees were affected. In the end he had to buy an expensive adjustable chair and all his aches and pains disappeared. If you have to spend a lot of time sitting, it really is important that your chair is adjustable so that it will support your body. It is a false economy to buy inexpensive or even expensive but badly designed chairs. Aches and pains and back problems make people miserable and bad tempered and unable to work properly – bosses please note.

If sitting on the floor is not easy, you can start with your back supported against a wall or sofa. Once you have developed a bit more strength and don't need so much support, try using your hands to prop you up. Always loosely fist your hands and don't press into the fingertips as this puts too much strain into the finger joints. Keep the elbows bent and don't lean back hunching your shoulders. You must work on these muscles to get them going after all this neglect. When you really work on your back muscles they will ache. This is a good ache from below the shoulders to the waist, so keep it up for a short while. As you work on these muscles it will disappear.

Sitting on the floor and getting the back straight

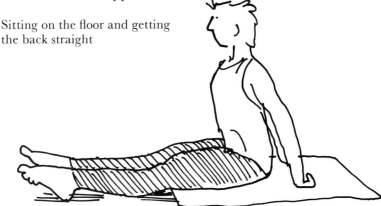

I have brought in these back muscles now because of their relevance to the forward movement of the body in the extension of the leg stretches. This may sound complicated when out of context with the exercises, but I can put that right.

SITTING WITH THE SOLES OF THE FEET TOGETHER
(Chart Ex. 53)

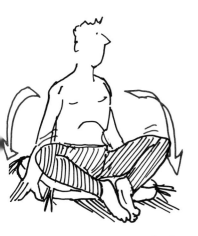

Sitting with the soles of the feet together, knees pressing down to open inside thigh and groin

Sit with the soles of your feet together and your back as straight as you can. (Sit against the wall if you need to or prop up with your arms.) Now where are your knees? Up round your ears? You need a cushion or folded towel under your bottom to lift you. This will help straighten your back too. Now press your knees down towards the floor. Hold, then release. Feel the stretch on the inside thigh and into the groin. Every time you stretch on the inside thigh you are pulling down on the outside thigh. Try to open up on the inside but don't force it. Remember everyone is formed differently so some people's thighs will just fall open easily while others may never get down very far. Get your feet in as close as you can without your back giving. It is more important to get the back up at this stage than to get the feet in close; this will come as you loosen up. Once you have done some slow down-presses with the knees, try bouncing them out gently.

Now let's work on your back. At first it may not move, so you will need your hands behind you. Then try letting go and resting your hands on your ankles. Do not hang on for dear life and try to pull yourself up with all the work in your arms and shoulders. Do not hold on to your feet either as you may pull the toes up, encouraging the feet to 'sickle'. Now try to pull your back up and through (pulling through means that your back not only lifts up straight but that the natural curve appears in the lower back).

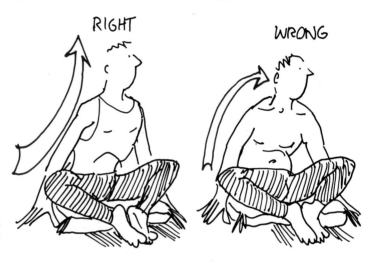

RIGHT   WRONG

Sitting with the soles of the feet together, getting the back right

This means that the ribs will lift in the front, opening up the space in the centre so that instead of folds of flesh there is a lifted space. Think how much better this is for the functioning of the digestive organs inside and for releasing the pressure on the spine as well as looking good. With the back lifted you should notice a difference in the tilt of your pelvis. Let your back round – pelvis rolls back. Then lift your back up – pelvis centres and you should be able to feel the sitting bones, (as in correct sitting). Pull the back through – pelvis tilts forwards and this will allow you to bring your body forwards with a straight back pivoting from the hips. Instead of trying to pull forwards from the waist as you would if your back was rounded and the pelvis dropped back.

Now you should begin to understand the importance of the back muscles in these exercises. There is no point in trying to bring your body forwards to increase the stretch in the backs of your thighs while your back is still rounded. All you will achieve is a hunched up, squashed up bundle heaving away at your ankles with more tension in your shoulders than stretch in your legs.

The French have an expression 'recourir pour mieux sauter', which means you must run again to jump better. So even if you felt you were going further with your back round, to get it right your back must be straight first.

SITTING WITH THE LEGS APART (Chart Ex. 54)

You stretched these muscles when you lay on your back with your legs apart. The difference here is that when you were lying down your back was supported and now, in the sitting position, your legs are supported and your back has got to do the work. Make sure your legs are equally apart: often you have one leg looser than the other, so bring this one in a bit or try to get the other one out until they are even. You will probably start to feel the stretch on the inside of your thigh at this stage. These are big muscles and they don't get much work in everyday life, so take it easy.

Now stretch your feet out as far as you can. This will help you to keep your knees down and will make your legs feel and look longer (flex them if you get cramp). The next stage is to get your back up. It helps if you can do this sitting sideways on to a mirror as this will help you see what you are feeling and confirm if it's right.

To get your arms out of the way, clasp your hands in front of you and straighten your arms, keeping your shoulders down. Lift your back up – when it is straight up you will feel your two sitting bones, this is your starting position. Without collapsing try to roll your pelvis back from this position by pulling in your tummy muscles. Be careful not to cheat by rounding your shoulders up and forwards to give the illusion of the rounded back. Your shoulders should remain straight and the top half of the body should stay as still as possible. Return to your starting position with the pelvis centred. Now try to pull your back through to tilt your pelvis forwards. (See also pelvic tilt page 15 Chart Ex. 1) This is very hard for most people and may take many months or even years to achieve. Don't be put off because something doesn't have instant results. All the time you are working your body, you are first counteracting natural degeneration (we begin to age from twenty years old) and secondly the unnatural stresses we put on the body (sitting in badly designed chairs for instance); add to

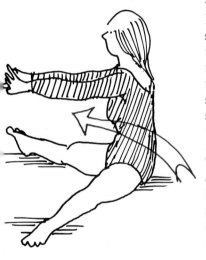

Pelvic rolling, sitting with legs apart roll pelvis back by pulling in tummy muscles

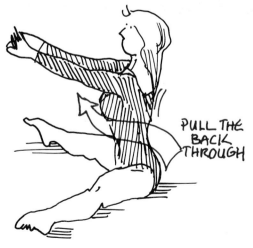

PULL THE BACK THROUGH

Pelvic rolling, sitting with legs apart pull back through to tilt pelvis forwards

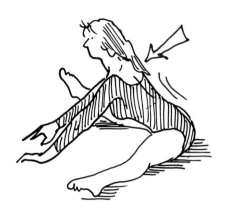

Sitting with legs apart, take
flat-backed body forwards

that the fact that your muscles have spent years getting into the
state they are in – so be patient even though results may not be
instant and spectacular, it all builds up. I did the splits for the
first time in my life at 33 and I have only just managed to get my
chest on the floor in the legs apart position. At least half the time
was spent trying to pull my back through. Once I had achieved
this, I could really get to work on going forwards. My inside thigh
was quite easy to stretch but I do have very tight hips. For those
of you who are constructed in the same way, don't be surprised
if you feel a 'pull' in your hip socket. Don't force it, there is a
large number of ligaments holding the thigh bone into the hip
socket. When these ligaments are loose and the inside thigh muscle
stretched, the legs can go straight out on either side of you (so
called double jointed). If your hips are that loose, do be careful
not to overstretch but to work very hard at keeping the outside
thigh muscles strong in order to hold the hip joint in place.

When you can really sit up straight in the starting position, you
can begin to take your flat-backed body forwards but don't do
the work with your arms and shoulders. This would just build
up negative tension and get you nowhere. You can only really
begin to take the body forwards when your pelvis can lead the
way with your back pulled through. I help people in my classes
to get the feel of this by placing one hand on the shoulder and the
other in the centre of the back. I then gently pull the shoulders
back as I push gently but firmly into the back. The hand in the
back really helps you feel where those muscles are and gives you
something to work on. Do remember that going forwards is a
progression and should only be done when the back, inside thighs
and hips have all reached a stage where they are prepared to go
further.

Once you've got the legs stretching, try flexing your feet. Be
careful that your knees don't pop up and don't let your legs roll
inwards at any stage. You can practise rotating your legs in the
hip socket from the starting position. Use your hands behind you

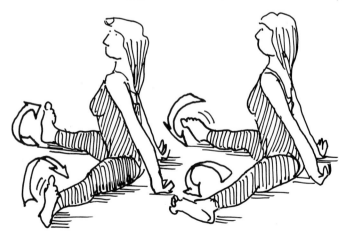

Thigh rotations

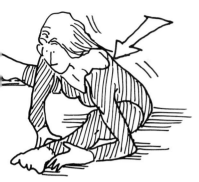

Inside thigh stretch, taking body forwards over one knee at a time

to give your back a rest. Relax the feet and start with one leg inwards and then outwards without your hip lifting off the ground. Next roll the other leg inwards and then outwards. Once you can rotate each leg separately try both legs together – you won't be able to lift your hip like this, so it may be harder. When your legs are apart always try to keep the knees facing straight up or roll the legs outwards to open up more.

When you start to stretch the inside thigh you may feel quite a strong pull by the knee. This is all right, but go gently, make sure your knees are facing upwards, and be careful that you are not feeling anything in the knee joint itself. If you do feel anything in the knee joint, bring your legs in a bit to lessen the stretch or get your knees checked if the pain continues.

Having achieved the best position you can try taking your body forwards over one leg at a time. Don't try to put your head on your knee with your shoulders round your ears in an attempt to reach your toes. Rather, keep your neck in line with the rest of your spine looking out towards your feet. If you place your arms out to the side of your body, this will stop you grabbing at your feet. Think of getting your chest on your thigh with the 'fold' at your hip not your waist.

After warming up the muscles with some long, slow stretches, try some gentle bounces to music. Make your own combination from the centre position to side, to side. How about ending up with your back flat and forwards, holding on to your flexed feet? Almost anything is possible if you give it time and practise regularly.

The last stretch is for the hamstrings and is usually thought of as 'touching your toes'. This unfortunate obsession with touching the toes causes many people to perform extraordinary contortions in order to achieve very little. The answer once again is that you will get nowhere until you approach the body position first. So let's start by testing the tightness of the hamstrings lying down.

HAMSTRING STRETCH (Chart Ex. 55)

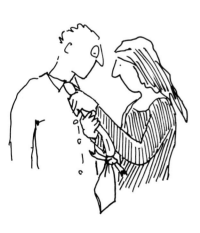

Before you get flat on your back, find a long belt or towel and place it beside you. Bend your knees into your chest and pull them into you to test the tightness of your back. Remember that if your back is tight it will contribute to the pull you will feel in your legs. It will also probably mean you have problems pulling your back through in the sitting position. But by lying down you can just concentrate on keeping it flat on the floor, which gives you more time to think about your legs.

Now hold the belt or towel over the soles of your feet and try straightening your legs up. By using the belt or towel you don't have to touch your toes in order to get your legs stretching and your back flat. Work on pulling up above the knees (quadriceps) to really straighten and stretch the back of your legs. I think this is a great stretch and often do it after a long hot bath when the muscles are relaxed and warm. It's especially good if you've spent all day on your feet as it helps drain the blood out of the bottom of your legs and reduces swelling in the ankles (unless this is caused by some more serious problem. Always check persistent ankle swelling). Don't forget to bend your knees into your chest to bring them down; don't try to bring them straight down (*see* tummy muscles). If your lower back is uncomfortable use a cushion under your pelvis as you did for the tummy muscle exercises.

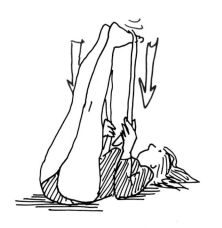

Hamstring stretch – lying on back and using towel

SITTING WITH LEGS STRAIGHT FORWARD (Chart Ex. 55)

Now sit up and try the same stretch, working on the back muscles at the same time. At first you will need the belt or towel to stop you hunching over your legs in an attempt to reach your toes. Apart from looking dreadful and building negative tension in your neck and shoulders you can end up with cramp in your tummy muscles, which I can assure you is not pleasant. If you do get cramp in your tummy muscles, stretch backwards to open them out.

Hamstring stretch – sitting with legs straight forward, using tie, with flat back

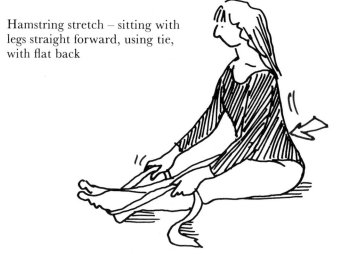

Put the belt or towel round your heels so that your feet can relax without flexing. Get your pelvis as lifted as possible, back straight, then pull forwards with elbows bent while holding on to either end of the belt. Make sure you're not taking the strain in your arms and shoulders; the belt or towel is an aid, you are not supposed to tear it in half.

When the stretch comes and the muscles begin to soften, you can try working without the belt. For some people just sitting up straight will be hard enough. If this is you, start against a wall or sofa to support your back. If you're feeling a stretch up the back of your legs, that's it – you're doing the exercise. Then progress to hands behind the back to prop you up (bent elbows, loose fist, shoulders down as before). Then back straight, no hands, no belt.

Time to tilt the pelvis! Hands are clasped, arms forward, back lifted, pelvis centred in starting position. Tummy pulls in, lower back rounds, pelvis tilts back. (This was the starting position for the tummy muscle curl-downs, remember?) Up to the starting position again and then lift your ribs to tilt the pelvis forwards and pull your back muscles through. Note that this starts the forward bend at the hips. If you try going forwards before your back pulls through, you will bend from the waist and it's back to the cramp in the tummy position.

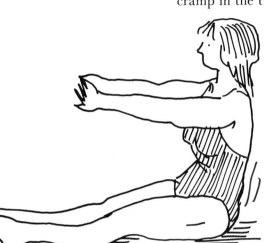 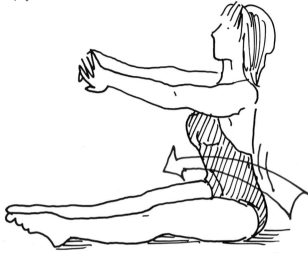

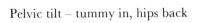

Pelvic tilt – tummy in, hips back

Pelvic tilt – back muscles pulled in, ribs lifted to tilt pelvis forward

Don't look at your knees. Be positive about where you are going. Your head will eventually end up way beyond your knees. Keep the neck in line with the rest of your spine. Rest your hands on your calves, ankles and eventually feet *without* rounding your shoulders up and forwards. Don't put your hands under your knees, though, as this will only encourage them to pop up off the floor.

Remember the knee exercise where you pulled up above the knees with the quadriceps and flexed your feet until the heels came up off the floor? Try the same thing with your body forwards – much stronger. If you're still using the belt, put it under the balls of your feet to achieve the same effect. While on the subject of knees again just check the position of your knees while your legs are straight out in front of you. They should face upwards and not turn in or out. If they are turning inwards you will probably find that your feet (one or both) are turning in. Try to get this straightened out. Unless there is a reason (birth defect, accident, etc.) this misalignment is purely muscular, probably originating from the hips and can be remedied with exercise. (Strengthening for the buttocks and back of the thighs will rotate the legs back outwards until they reach their correct position.)

Stretching one leg at a time, sit with your back straight and legs out in front of you; bend one leg in so that the sole of the foot rests on the inside of the thigh, be careful not to tuck the foot *under* your leg as this will encourage your knee to lift off the floor.

Take your body forwards over the straight leg, first with the foot stretched or relaxed then flexed. You can use the belt or towel if you need to; then change legs. You may find that one of your legs is tighter than the other and therefore needs extra stretching. Never stretch only one leg; stretch them both and then give the tighter one an extra stretch.

Remember that in order to really stretch muscle you must hold the stretch to sustain it. When you have put your body into the best position you can achieve and allowed the muscle to open out, try some loose bounces to music as this will always liven you up and make you feel you're really working.

Do always warm up your muscles before attempting any gigantic stretches such as the splits. I tore all the muscles up the back of my leg by trying this when not warm – I know I should have known better, but sometimes we have to learn by our own mistakes and this was a particularly painful one – muscle sounds like Velcro when it tears and it took eighteen months to heal. I was lucky my muscles were in good condition. If you tear unused muscles (which is more likely if they are hard and tight), the scar tissue sometimes never heals properly. So get stretching but do it with care and understanding. As I have explained, there is no point in aiming blindly for your toes until you have achieved certain preliminaries and understood the basic principles.

To bend forward towards your toes stand up. Start with your feet together (big toe joints and heels touching) with arms by your side. Pull up above your knees and bring your body forwards slowly with your back flat (pulling in your tummy). So you fold forward from the hips. When you can go no further with your back flat, relax down, arms hanging forwards, head free and roll the weight of your body forwards, towards the balls of your feet. At first you simply can't wait to come up out of this position but after a while you will find it marvellously relaxing, with the blood being helped to the head, the body loose and free. When your hands touch the floor, work them back towards the feet with the back of your hand on the floor. Eventually as the muscles stretch you will fold in two. To come up out of this position always bring the head up first followed by the shoulders and top of the back so that you come up with a flat back. Use your tummy muscles to help you do this. The back is much better protected in this position. When you come up with a round back, with the head coming up last, you are having to carry the weight of your head in the back (in the same way you used the weight of the head in the first neck exercise), so make sure you understand what you are doing and use the body with care.

If you are given bounces forward to stretch the back of the

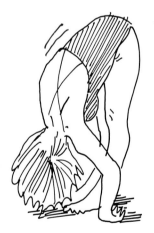

Forwards bend towards toes, standing – feet together, arms by your sides, fold body from the hips legs, make sure that you have already done some gentler warm up first especially if your legs are very tight.

There are flat back bounces and round back bounces which are often done with music. Feet should be apart. Flat back bounces are with hand flat on the floor. Round back bounces are pulling in the tummy, rounding your back and pulling your head and arms through your legs. Not good for weak backs. Nor are flat back forward bounces good for weak backs as all the strain is taken at the fulcrum which, in this case, is the lower back. Stretching out your hamstring so that you can fully straighten your legs will totally change their shape. Instead of short bulky muscle in the thigh the strength will be distributed along the full length of the muscles, giving them a long smooth shape.

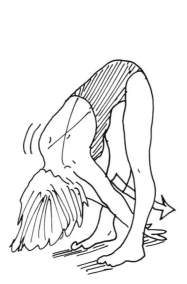

Round back bounces – feet apart, tummy pulled in, pull head and arms through legs

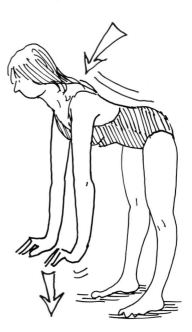

Flat back bounces – feet apart

7 Calves and Tendons

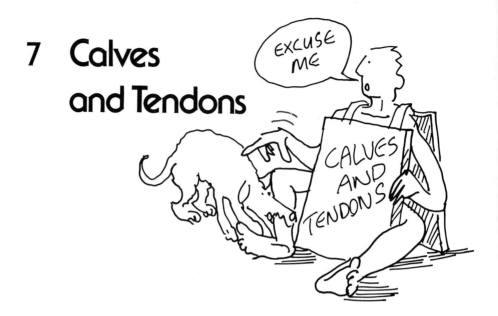

This chapter deals with the lower part of the leg. The main bulk of the calf which gives it its shape is called the *gastrocnemius*. It is formed by two bundles of muscle which are joined to the end of the thigh bone (femur) at the knee and then unite into a long tendon which ends up at the heel. This is what we call the Achilles tendon. The other big calf muscle lies behind the *gastrocnemius* and is called the *soleus*; this also attaches to the Achilles tendon. There are also muscles which control the movements of the feet, ankles and toes.

Many people have unbelievably tight calves and this puts an immense strain on the Achilles tendon.

To understand this you must briefly look at the construction of a muscle. Muscles are made up of short fibres. These are held together in bundles by fibrous tissue which narrows down to form the tendon. It is the tendons which attach to bones or other fibrous tissue and the placing of this attachment is what determines the movement made. When a muscle contracts, the fibres shorten and this will flex a joint. When they stretch, this will extend a joint. In simple joint movements they work in pairs as I explained with the arm movements.

The tendon is not elastic like the muscle because it is fibrous tissue. Where you have a long tendon, therefore, it is very import-

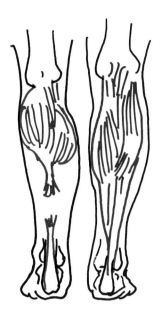

Showing the *gastrocnemius* and *soleus* muscles – left: broken tendon caused by extra strain on muscles

ant to keep the stretchy part of the muscle in really good condition. Maybe you can walk around for years with tight calves but one day you will put that extra tug on the muscle, perhaps on the tennis court or during some other exertion which you are not trained up for, and snap! The muscle cannot give and stretch, so the hard fibrous tissue of the tendon breaks. The problem is made worse because the muscle end of the tendon shoots up into the calf, so that the tighter the muscle the harder it is to pull it down again in order to pin the two halves of tendon together again. As you can imagine, this is very painful and involves surgery and weeks with your leg in plaster.

CALF STRETCH (Chart Ex. 23)

To avoid broken tendons, let's start by testing the tightness of your calves. Find a wall or table or chair back to rest your hands on. Step forwards with your left foot, bending the knee. Make sure it doesn't push out beyond the heel and that the weight is on the outside of the foot. Take the right leg well behind you without your

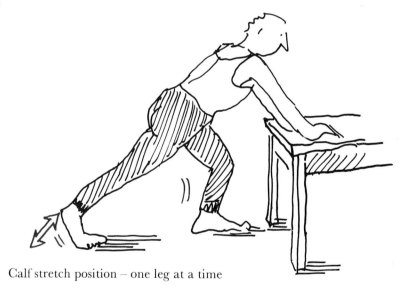

Calf stretch position – one leg at a time

foot turning out. Keep your body upright and don't immediately bring your shoulders round your ears leaning all your weight forwards. Keeping your bottom tucked in and not sticking out behind you will help this. Now push your right heel down towards the ground and then release it. Just keep pushing down and releasing until your heel can stay down on the floor. Then hold it. Try to keep your weight back into your right heel so that you don't put any strain into the left knee. You will soon know how tight your calf is by the strong pull up the back of your right calf. Change legs and test the left leg in the same way. Right knee bend, foot flat on the floor; left leg straight back resting on the ball of the foot and then pressing down and releasing, ending with a long press down.

As the muscle stretches change the position slightly to get more of a stretch. Starting again with the right leg back (it is not important which leg you start with as long as you always work both legs, it just makes it easier for me to explain), take it as far back as you can and this time keep the heel on the floor. Bend the left knee and rest on the ball of the left foot, keeping the knee bent. Don't get too far away from whatever you're supporting your hands on otherwise your bottom will stick out. Also, don't turn your back foot out as this will completely negate the stretch and you will be cheating yourself. Now push forwards with your right hip, still keeping your body and leg in one line. Try quick pushes in time to music and then a slow one, holding for about eight counts. Then change legs and work on the left leg in the same way. You could end by working both legs together leaning the body forwards. But be careful to keep the body straight!

These exercises not only test the tightness of the calves, they also stretch them out as you will have felt. I do them every day. Kitchen surfaces or office desks make an excellent place to rest your hands and everyone has the odd couple of minutes to spare during the day, so why not use them to stretch your calves. The more you can incorporate exercises into your everyday life, the less of a chore they become and the more likely you are to do them.

Stretching the calves is particularly important before you participate in any kind of sport where you will be using your legs.

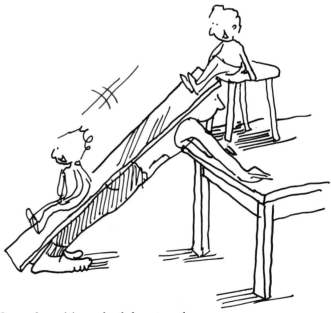

Calf stretch position – both legs together

Tennis, running, jogging, dancing, etc., are all going to rely heavily on action in the calves. It is the *gastrocnemius* muscle which gives us our quick springing movements, while the *soleus* which lies behind it is used more to stabilise us when standing. Here is a quick stretch you can do to warm the muscles up before a run or a game: put your feet and legs together and bend your knees; rest your hands on your knees and then push down with gentle bounces, knees out over the feet. This should not put any strain on your knees. If your knees are that weak, you should check before doing any kind of sport as this would probably put too much pressure on them anyway. In the same position (knees and feet together) try a variation of this by cycling the knees first to the right, bending as you push forward and straightening as the knees come back. Then circle to the left, making sure that you really bend the knees to get a good stretch on the calves as you go forwards.

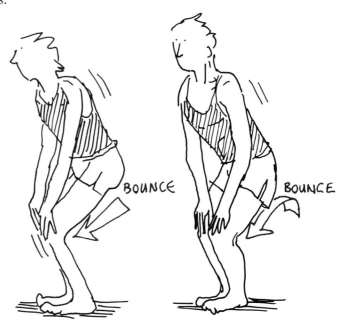

Calf stretch exercise – hands on knees, gentle push-down bounces

Calf stretch exercise variation – circling knees to right then left as you bounce

The last calf stretch I would recommend is in fact a yoga position, the 'dog' pose. I think it is rather a pleasant way to stretch. It gives your arms and back a lovely stretch too. Lie on your tummy on the floor and put your hands under your shoulders with the elbows bent up by the side of your body. Bend your toes back so that you are resting on the balls of your feet. Straighten your arms and push your bottom up into the air and pushing your weight back into your heels. Your back and arms should be straight with your head between your arms, your neck and in line

The 'dog' pose

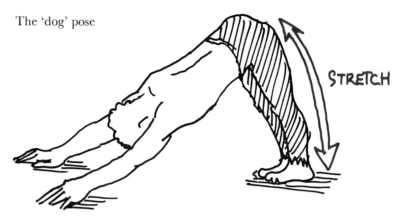

STRETCH

with the rest of your spine. Don't alter the position of your hands or feet, just stay there letting the stretch come until you can get your heels further into the floor (they probably won't go down at first). To come down from this position lower the hips into the floor bending and supporting with the arms. As well as stretching them it is also important to keep the calves strong. Strengthening the calves will also improve the shape and as the muscle contracts and releases it will help push the blood up through the muscle fibres. This is particularly important in the lower part of the leg as it is the furthest part of the body from the heart and it also has to contend as does everything else with the pull of gravity. The body has two main kinds of blood vessel: the veins and the arteries. These then divide up into a web and end up as fine vessels called capillaries which feed the cells and take away their waste products. Arteries are strong, thick elastic-walled tubes which take the freshly oxygenated blood from the heart out around the body to the capillaries. The strong pumping action of the heart pushes the blood into the arteries. With the exception of the arteries which supply the brain, this flow is helped by the force of gravity.

The veins are thinner-walled vessels which take the 'used' blood from the capillaries back to the lungs where the carbon dioxide is again exchanged for oxygen. Other waste products are also collected from the cells; these are mainly uric and lactic acid which are given off by the muscles as the by-product of the energy they release when working. Because the veins are having to work against gravity most of the time and the blood is having to run uphill (again with the exception of the veins from the head to the heart), there are valves in the veins. As the blood is moved along the veins, helped by the suction action of breathing and muscular contraction in the extremities, these valves open and close to stop the blood running back. If these valves become impaired the blood will 'pool' and the veins become permanently dilated. These are called varicose veins. There are many causes of varicose veins. Sometimes they are hereditary and sometimes they are worsened by excessive standing or pregnancy, or just weak muscles.

Working the calf muscles will help prevent varicose veins since, by contracting the muscles, you help squeeze the blood up through them. If the muscle is permanently tight, though, this makes it harder for the blood to force its way through the constricting fibres. It is again important therefore to always release (stretch out) the muscles after contracting them. If you have varicose veins already, do check with your doctor about exercise as this will depend on his treatment.

STRENGTHENING THE CALVES (Chart Ex. 22)

Find a wall, table or chair back on which to rest your fingers; do not cling on, but try to 'feel' your balance. Put your toes and heels together so that the insides of your feet are touching. Note whether your big toes are pointing away from each other, forming a 'V' shape; if they are turn to the next chapter for the remedy.

Now rise up onto the balls of your feet. Pull up above your knees so that your legs are straight and tuck your bottom firmly underneath you and pull in your tummy to centre your pelvis. Just try bringing your hands above your head without your shoulders coming up and see if you can balance. Are you weaving a bit? Well don't worry, hold on again and concentrate on the calf exercise at first. You should be standing correctly, neck long, chest lifted, shoulders relaxed, pelvis centred, knees straight. Now rise up onto the balls of your feet again with the heels as high off the floor as you can get them – this contracts the calf. Then release by

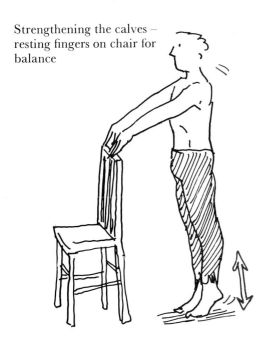

Strengthening the calves – resting fingers on chair for balance

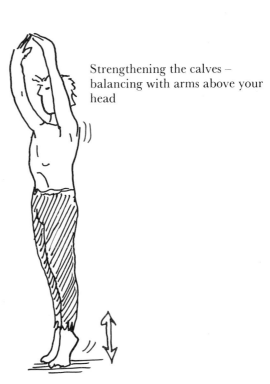

Strengthening the calves – balancing with arms above your head

taking the heels halfway down to the ground and then pop up again. Keep going up and down (knees straight, remember) until you feel the calves tighten. If they were very tight to start with, then only do a few of these at first just to get the muscle fibres going. To break up tight muscle fibres that have become stuck together you must work them in every way and as much as possible. Muscles respond to work, that's what they are made for. When you finish this exercise – which should be before your calves go into spasm, so don't overdo it at first – ALWAYS DO ONE OF THE STRETCHES TO FINISH. You should also make sure you stretch out your calves if you wear high heels as they are holding your calves in a permanent contraction up on the balls of your feet, which brings me back to the balance of the body.

Remember the balancing pencil? (See page 18.) If you stand a pencil up on its end it will balance, but if you tip the pencil slightly it will fall down. When the pencil is upright the centre of gravity is straight through the middle of it. We are far more clever than a pencil because we are bendy and not rigid, so that if gravity pulls more on one side than the other we can immediately form a compensatory curve to counteract it. As we have seen in previous chapters, if these compensatory curves are used too frequently they become a habit and eventually a permanent feature of our posture. So it is very important that we always come back to the centred position. Balancing on the balls of the feet is a very good way to practise this.

If you've got a mirror handy, do use it as many people feel 'wrong' at first when they correct their position. Stand sideways on to the mirror to see best what is happening. Have your wall,

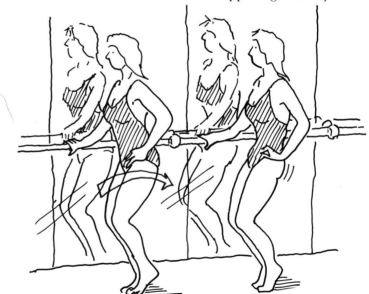

Tilting the pelvis backwards and forwards to find centre for balance

table or chair back handy to give you confidence to start with. Toes, heels and legs together, rise up onto the balls of the feet as you did in the calf strengthener. Bend your knees and try a few pelvic tilts, releasing first to let your pelvis tilt forward (bottom out) and then pulling in your tummy to bring your pelvis back with your buttocks tightening at the same time. End of a forward tilt, tummy in and tight bottom. Now straighten your legs and pull up above your knees. With your centre strong (tummy and buttocks tucked under) you should have a lifted body. The mistake most people make is to over arch their backs and push their chins forwards. A lot of people (including me) feel very strange in the correct position at first. It made me feel rather like a gorilla with my top half so unaccustomedly forward. This is why the mirror is so invaluable because you can *see* when you are in the right position even if it *feels* wrong.

Lift your arms and round them above your head. You are now balancing. Don't wobble about and lean back; keep your heels together. If the heels come apart persistently this is due to weakness in the outside ankle and I am dealing with that next. While you are up on the balls of your feet and balancing, try a few calf strengtheners by taking the heels up and half way down. Don't forget to stretch the calves afterwards.

ANKLE EXERCISES (Chart Ex. 17)

Sit down again on your chair or stool. Place your feet slightly forwards and apart, just beyond hip width. Now let your knees drop inwards so that your inside thighs come together.

We will start by working on the outside ankle muscle because it is normally the weakest. That's why when you twist your ankle it goes outwards and why your heels came apart in the balance. Turn your feet out without your knees parting. If you find this rather confusing at first, try putting your fisted hand between your knees to give you something to grip on (don't let your body slump, though). Knees in, feet out, now lift your little toes up towards the outside of your knees. The foot should turn as it lifts. Really try to keep the foot turning out and get everything but the heel lifting off the ground.

You may be surprised to feel this pulling all the way up your lower leg. This is because the muscle (*peroneus longus*) attaches all the way up to your knee and ends in the middle of the foot.

To work the inside ankle keep the knees in the same position but swivel your feet inwards so that you look pigeon-toed. Now lift the big toes up towards the inside of your knees. This will feel much harder as you are working with the stronger muscle (*tibialis anterior*). You will feel these working up your legs as they are also long muscles.

Do your lifts both on the inside and outside, at varying speeds. Start off slowly and then build up to fast lifts.

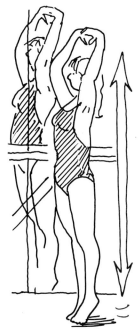

Balancing with pelvis centred

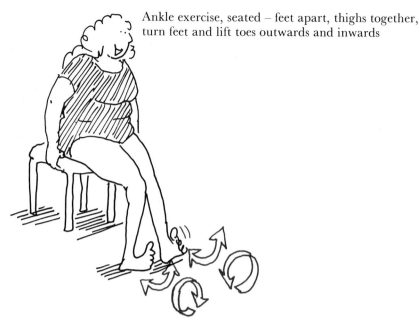

Ankle exercise, seated – feet apart, thighs together, turn feet and lift toes outwards and inwards

Once you have mastered the outside and inside lifts try combining them. This gives you a lovely sweeping movement which takes you halfway through an ankle circle.

Lift the feet to the outside and then sweep them down to the floor and lift them inwards, then back through the floor to lift on the outside again. Keep this movement smooth and rhythmical but don't allow it to send you to sleep – you need to concentrate on this one to make sure you really do pull up at each side.

Full ankle circles are also very beneficial as they keep the joints mobile as well as working on the muscles. When you circle your foot *inwards*, the emphasis is on the *outside* ankle muscle (so more of these). When you circle the foot *outwards* you are working more on the *inside* ankle muscle. Ankle circles can be done at any time that you are sitting with a moment to spare.

I would just like to put in a bit about aerobics here. I have hinted at running, jumping and other energetic activities in previous chapters, but now I feel is the time to start pushing the subject!

I loathed gym at school and I hated games – I still do, I am temperamentally unsuited to games as I'm not a good loser. I even cheat at snakes and ladders with my kids! Tennis was all right, but I was not allowed to play after I slipped the disc in my neck as overarm shots put a tremendous strain on that area. Anyway, it was only really a good way for meeting boys! Until a few years ago the idea of getting sweaty didn't enter my mind. But as my body improved through gentle exercise (remember I really was in horrendous shape having done NOTHING for the first 27 years of my life) I felt that I wanted to extend it more.

My marriage was breaking up and my children were at school full-time, so I went back to work. All the classes I had been doing had been during the day and so suddenly here I was sitting at a desk and driving around London all day with my body disintegrating fast. It was then that a friend suggested the Dance Centre. Apart from grooving around on various dance floors, I had never 'danced' in my life. Packed like sardines in a steaming studio the music started and we went through a series of warm-up exercises. So far, so good; I was well trained and my body easily adapted to the exercises. Second part of the class was the routine. What a disaster! What was a step ball change anyway? And why did everyone change direction just when I'd got the hang of going the other way? All I knew when I came out was that I may have been trampled on in the back row but I couldn't wait to get back! I persisted. The studios all had a mirror down one wall and viewing windows on the other. I soon discovered my place at the back in the corner furthest from the windows and the mirror. When you were really good you were up front concentrating on your own image and in full view of anyone who cared to watch. I took two or three classes a night, three nights a week, until I picked up the basic steps sufficiently to graduate to somewhere near the middle of the middle; but to this day I'm not quick at picking up routines. I love dancing and the music and the feeling of having used my body totally. It also had a marvellous effect on me mentally.

All marriage break-ups are traumatic. It affects the children and everyone gets hurt, feels a sense of failure, guilt, regret, bitterness and many other mixed emotions. Physically working my body to its limits helped me to cope with these stresses. I cannot emphasise enough the mind–body connection. The more you sit and brood over your problems, the bigger they loom in your mind. The more depressed you get, the more difficult it is to make a first move.

One thing I discovered from those dance classes, was the importance of music. Once the music starts it gets into your body and compels it to move. Even the ankle exercises done sitting down go with a swing to music.

Now there are available in Britain the workout classes from California. These are non-stop stretch and aerobic exercises. So, if you are like me and always one step behind in the dance routine, you can go through a whole class of rhythmical exercises. Do apply all the principles you have learned in this book, though. If the teacher is good she will keep an eye on her class, not spend her time looking at herself in the mirror. If you're given leg raising exercises for your tummy and you feel them only in your back, don't do them. Substitute another exercise. You're doing the class for the good of *your* body.

Then there are aerobic classes which are sometimes incorporated in the workout class. These involve a combination of non-stop runs on the spot and jumps. I always include some of these in my Hardworking Bodywork classes and although there were groans at first people soon began to feel the benefit.

I also teach a purely aerobic class. This consists of at least twenty minutes jumping. I started with a few curious pupils including Mary. Mary is in her thirties and has a wonderful lean body. She plays tennis and thought she was quite fit. After the first three minutes jumping she was walking around wheezing. After five weeks of classes (one aerobic and one hardworking bodywork class a week) she was jumping full time and feeling great. You do get a high from physical exertion, and for me jumping to music is sheer fun, and it's non-competitive. But you must prepare your body first – this is *keeping* fit.

In the summer I like running and jogging in the park but I still have the music in my head to put rhythm in my feet. I'm not too keen on running in the snow and rain, but this is my personal preference so don't you be put off! Whatever you choose, though, to get your heart and lungs going there are a few vital bits of advice that should not be ignored . . .

You *must* warm up before you begin. It's all very well buying the new shoes and track suit and just opening the front door and expecting to dash out and run for miles. The body must be stretched to start with.

WARMING UP AND WARMING DOWN

Start off with shoulder circles, then develop these into arm swings to loosen the joints. (See p. 29)

Follow these with some body twists with your hands resting on your shoulders and elbows lifted.

Do keep your pelvis centred and your legs firm all the time you are moving the top half of your body. Next, some side bends and then some forward bends to stretch your hamstrings. (See p. 71)

Do keep your bottom firm all the time you are moving the top half of your body. Next, some side bends and some forward bends to stretch your hamstrings.

If your lower back is weak, rest your leg on a table top to stretch your hamstrings rather than touching your toes standing up.

Stretch the quadriceps standing on one leg and pulling the other leg up behind you. (page 81) Stretch the inside thigh by stretching one leg out sideways and bending the other knee so you feel a pull on the inside thigh of the straight leg. Keep your legs turned out.

Most important of all stretch the calves. Try to hold all stretches to give the muscles time to open up.

Finally try a few quick runs on the spot with short rests in between to start the heart beat increasing, then off you go.

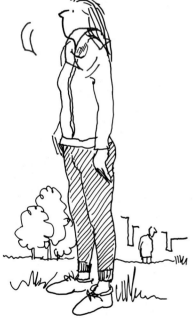

Warming up and warming down exercises – shoulder circles

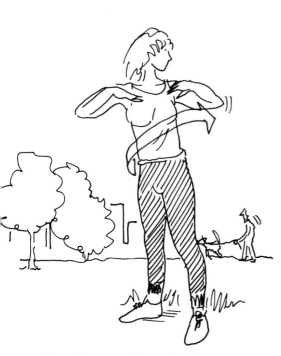

Warming up and warming down exercises – body twists, hands on shoulders

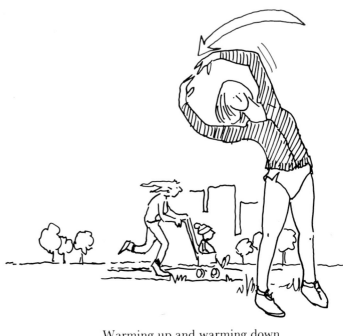

Warming up and warming down exercises – side bends

Warming up and warming down exercises – running on the spot

Warming up and warming down – stretch quadriceps standing on one leg

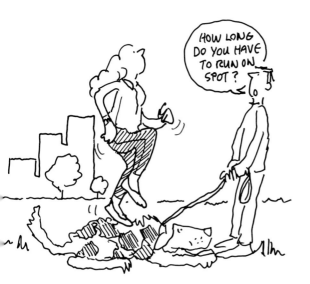

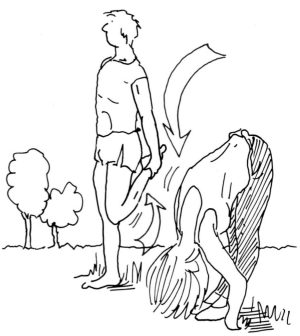

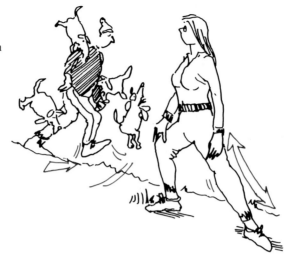

Warming up and warming down exercises – forward stretch to stretch hamstrings

Try not to stop suddenly at whatever you are doing. If it is running, pace yourself so that when you feel tired you slow down and walk for a bit. This will stop you exhausting yourself on your first attempt and putting yourself off for life. This applies in an aerobics class too. If you simply can't keep up the jumping at first, just jog or walk on the spot but KEEP YOUR LEGS MOVING.

When you have finished your vigorous warming up exercise it is ESSENTIAL THAT YOU WARM DOWN. There is a tremendous increase in circulation while you are leaping about and the leg muscles are literally contracting and pushing that blood up to the heart against gravity. In turn the heart is pumping the blood back down into the legs. If the muscles suddenly relax the blood 'pools'.

First of all slow your movement gently down by decreasing your activity; this gives the heart time to adjust its beat. Follow this with the same stretches and body looseners that you warmed up with. This will also help you prevent stiffness which is caused by the waste products produced by increased energy levels. These waste products which, if not flushed away, will build up between the muscle fibres causing them to 'stick' together instead of moving freely.

A word of warning, don't eat anything before you exercise or you will feel terrible! Apart from making you feel sick it can also cause cramp. You never know, with your new energy level you may not feel hungry afterwards either. Feeling sick during an exercise can also be lack of fitness, so stop.

Lastly, do make sure that you're properly dressed. A track suit to warm up in and to put on for warming down. Loose comfortable clothes to allow you movement, and good shoes. Good shoes are very important and are really worth investing in even though they are expensive. Make sure that there is plenty of room for your toes to spread out in them and that they are wide enough. You should also be able to wear fairly thick socks inside them. They should have thick insoles and should not have a high tab up the Achilles tendon. The next chapter will help you understand more about your feet and how to care for them.

8 Down to Earth

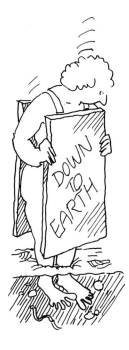

Your feet are what put you in touch with the earth. We walk, run, and jump on them. We cram them into an amazing assortment of shoes and at the end of the day we put them up. And that's about as much thought as we give them!

Yet in Biblical times they saved their most precious oils to anoint the feet and in a special kind of foot massage called reflexology we find that the soles of the feet correspond to the vital parts of the body. So why do we pay so little regard to such an important part of us?

From our first tottering step our tiny feet are encased in shoes. Certainly I would not recommend walking down the streets of any city with bare feet, and shoes and boots do keep our feet warm in winter. But I think we spend far too little time with bare feet. Badly fitting shoes can deform the feet for life and cause untold pain and loss of mobility in later life. Shoes are one of the items of clothing I really think it is worth spending money on *especially* for children. Young growing feet need room to move and this includes the socks as well as the shoes. Too small socks can cause as many problems as restrictive shoes.

Then there are high heels. I would *never* buy a child a pair of shoes with heightened heels. They are bad enough when the foot has stopped growing. At this point I'd better stop being holier

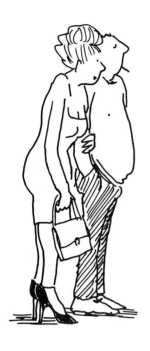

than thou and confess that at 5ft 1in. I feel best in a pair of high heels! They make your legs look longer and sexier and I guess that if they are in fashion then, like everyone else, I want to wear them.

Let me explain what they do, not only to your feet but also to the rest of your posture. Have you ever seen this lady before? Can you see what the high heels have done to her body? They have thrown her whole weight forwards and into the ball of her foot, causing her bottom to stick out! This does not look sexy. And the more cramped the foot becomes, the more mincing the walk. On the serious side imagine the damage this is causing.

Any shoe that squashes the toes, and this applies to flat ones too, is going to squeeze them together. As the big toe turns inwards the bunion bone protrudes. Remember putting your toes and heels together in the last chapter? Were you the one with the 'V' shaped toes? If you had any one of your toes removed, it would drastically affect your balance and you would have to learn to walk again. Screwing up your toes affects your balance, but because it happens over a number of years the body has time to compensate. You may well remain standing but what sort of shape are your toes in? Many people are revolted by their feet and taking a look at them I'm not surprised! Old gnarled joints and hard skin and blisters are hardly a lovely sight. But feet can be beautiful. I am not a foot fetishist myself, but I do feel that we are denying a part of our body the attention it deserves.

Back to the misalignment caused by high heels. Look at what happens to the ankle joint and how this affects the knees. And what about the tilt of the pelvis? Can you now understand why high heels cause bad backs?

I'm not asking anyone to give up high heels completely, although if you have a severe lower back problem they will only make it worse. I'm trying to point out what happens when you wear high heels and I am now going to give some practical suggestions to counteract their effect. By the way, high heels are anything over two inches, so this includes a certain amount of men's shoes too!

First, try not to wear them for too long at a time especially if you are going to have to walk or stand for long hours. The lower the heels the better for these activities and you can still find pretty shoes in this style. Have bare feet as often as possible to allow the toes to move freely. Always stretch out the calves after wearing high heels to prevent them tightening up permanently.

If your feet are sore and swollen, try putting them in ice cold water to take the swelling down. Or alternate between a bucket of very cold water and a bucket of hot water to increase the circulation. Put your feet up to help drain away the swelling. If you have any kind of persistent swelling or water retention (oedema) rather than just tired feet, always check with your

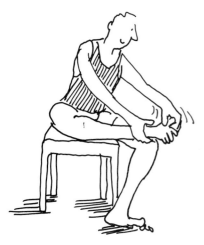

Foot massage – rest foot on other leg

doctor. Avoid strong diuretics as these put a terrible strain on your kidneys.

Shoes should support the feet and allow movement of the toes. They should fit properly both in length and width and they should be comfortable. A reputable shoe shop will always make sure of these things before you buy. The rest is up to you.

Try massaging your feet. There is nothing more relaxing. Obviously it is even better if you can get someone to do this for you. Here are some ways to massage your feet.

Sit resting your foot on your other leg. Start by separating the toes. Gently pull the little and big toes away from each other so that the inner toes can spread. Now work with your thumbs over the bottom toe joints (nearest your foot), especially the bunion bone. This may be painful so be very gentle. Try and open up the spaces between the toes by interlocking your fingers between each toe. Then work your way along each toe from the foot outwards. Use your thumb and forefinger to stroke along the toe and work over the joints. Put some cream on your foot and massage it in, covering the whole area right up to the ankle and around the heel. Pay special attention to the sole of the foot.

I am not myself a practitioner of reflexology but I have shown you the foot chart anyway because I think it is so fascinating.

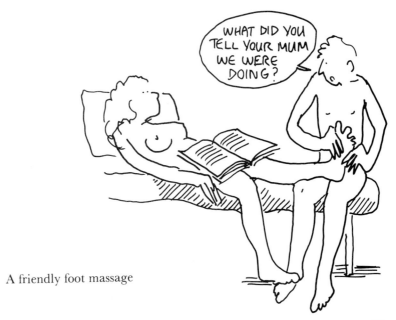

A friendly foot massage

It is obviously much better if someone can do this for you. To massage the foot in this way, you use your thumbs working horizontally across the foot. Don't press too hard as some areas may be very painful. Don't be too light either or you will just tickle the foot. The painful areas will usually feel grainy under the skin. Don't work too long on the feet at first, about five to ten minutes.

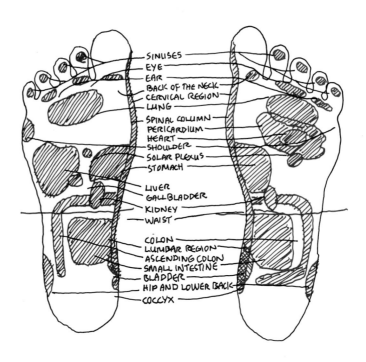

Reflexology foot chart

Start with the big toe on the right foot and move along the toes massaging the zones for the sinuses, the eyes, the ears, the bronchia, the lungs and the liver. Be careful not to overdo the liver, this could cause diarrhoea! Be careful to always massage the intestinal zone clockwise to correspond with the peristaltic wave. This is the rhythmical wave that carries the food through the digestive system and which must not be disturbed.

Through finding the grainy and painful areas of the foot, you can discover which parts of the body are not functioning at their optimum – maybe as a result of a past illness or as a sign of something going wrong and to be watched for the future. Remember, though, diagnosis is for doctors and not for amateur guesswork. Reflexology may sort out minor problems and can be used to relieve everyday aches and pains. Its practice is as old as acupuncture and acupressure.

A FOOTNOTE ON BALLS!

If you don't have a friend handy to massage your feet, all you need is a ball! This is one of the most relaxing things you can do for your body. Just slip off your shoes and place the ball under your foot – if you've got two balls and are sitting down, you can do both feet at once!

Sitting down is the best position, but one foot at a time standing will do. Now all you have to do is roll that ball about under your foot – it's so simple!

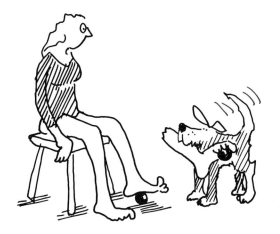

Foot massage with a ball

Cover the whole area of the foot right up under the toes, round the tips of the toes, over the ball of the foot, all round the instep, along the outside edges and all around the heel. Any order will do; just go on rolling the ball up and down and from side to side. Don't miss out the sensitive parts and check where they correspond to your reflexology chart.

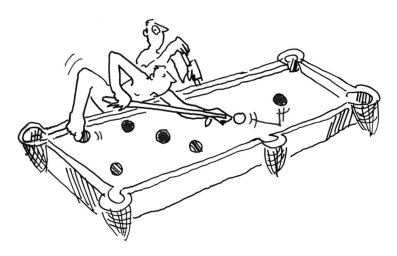

You will soon discover the right pressure to apply. Too much or too little and the ball shoots off! I use old squash balls as I find these a good size and consistency. Try tennis balls or the dog's ball – footballs, in spite of their name, are too big! Massage the foot for about three to five minutes and then stand up. You will find that the whole side of your body has softened and loosened up, so it is not just your foot which is affected and which benefits.

FOOT EXERCISES (Chart Ex. 21)

Here are two foot exercises which affect the arches of the foot. Sitting with your legs hip-width apart, feet forwards but with

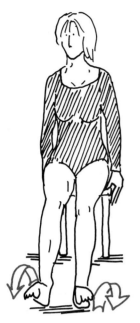

Foot exercise –
gripping with your toes

your knees still bent, turn your feet up towards your shins, then grip the balls of your feet with your toes and then release. Squeeze and release at various speeds, spread your toes out to finish, then wiggle them. I'm not sure why, but some people feel sick when they do this exercise. I have yet to find the official explanation but try and work through this. It is important to keep this first meta-tarsal arch lifted, and the more you use the muscles the more any blockages should loosen. My toes were in a terrible state – I have broken three of them at various stages in my life. This exercise has helped them enormously; it has given them strength and I can even see the 'knuckles' on my feet when I squeeze my toes over.

The second exercise is for the main arch of the foot – the instep. This is a vital arch. Think of the brickwork of an arched window. There is a centre stone which maintains the arch and if this goes everything collapses. Apply this to the structure of the foot and you should have an idea of what flat feet do to you. The whole weight of the body totally misdistributes, as we have seen before. Either use a mirror or lean forwards to watch this exercise when you first try to perform it. Most people simply can't get the message through to the muscle at first so you need the visual feedback to build on.

Start with your feet flat on the floor (you can turn them out if you are looking at them in a mirror, so that you see the arch). Now press the pads of your toes lightly into the floor to stop them

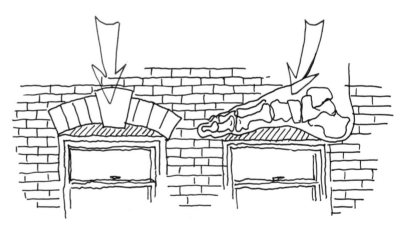

curling up, then draw the ball of your feet in towards your heel, shortening and pulling up the arches.

Nothing happening, or just the toes scrunging up? Try this: place a fat book under your toes, press down on your toes and pull up on your arch. The book will stop your toes curling under and give you more chance to concentrate on your arch. This exercise can take time to achieve. Look for any sign of movement in the arch and work on it. Once you have mastered it you will be able to contract your arches at any speed even standing up inside your shoes.

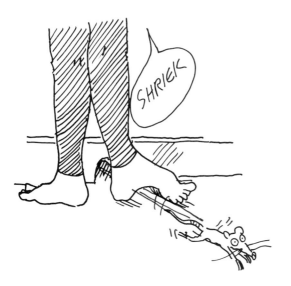

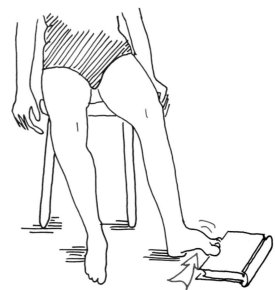

Foot exercise to strengthen arches, drawing ball of foot in towards heel

Foot exercise to strengthen arches, using fat book under toes

Some people's feet just spread with age. Women's feet often spread after having a baby. This is because hormones are released in pregnancy to soften the ligaments to allow the pelvis to open for birth. The hormones affect all the ligaments, including those in the feet. Add to this the increased weight and your feet can gain half a size. Mine did for years but this exercise brought them back to their original size again.

Some people take a lot of tension in their feet and may walk around with their toes all screwed up and their arches permanently contracted in their shoes. This kind of tension is just as bad as tight necks and shoulders and will affect your whole outlook in the same way. Tightness and the pain it causes make you ratty and bad tempered, so sort out the muscles to sort out the mood. Exercise gently on tight toes but exercise them nevertheless. Lots of massage and care and make sure that you are wearing proper fitting shoes. There is nothing more exhausting than painful feet. Just recap on Chapter I dealing with correct standing. Remember the tripod points of the foot. Weight should be felt in the heels, balls of the feet and along the outside of the feet (because the arch is lifted), and the toes should be left long.

One last word on feet. There are certain nerve endings in the foot which stimulate a reflex in the body which makes us stand erect. This is called the planter reflex. Every time we walk or run this reflex is stimulated, which keeps us standing upright. Old people sometimes start to shuffle; this does not stimulate the planter reflex so that the body begins to curve forwards. If this is happening to you or someone you know, get them to sit down and just stamp their feet on the ground, if they are too weak to do it standing up. The planter reflex also needs stimulating if you have to spend long periods in bed. Think of how weak the muscles become from not being used and how droopy you are when you first get up. Keep the planter reflex stimulated by 'stamping' the feet on the end of the bed. Put a board there, preferably, and don't go mad at it. Try to keep all your muscles moving (within reason if you are bed-ridden). Even small movements count. Then you will be ready to spring to your feet when you are well again.

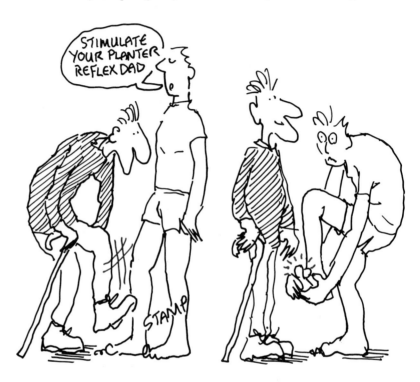

Keep the planter reflex stimulated by stamping feet

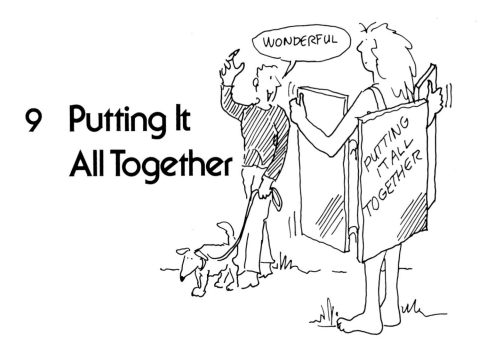

9 Putting It All Together

This last chapter puts all the exercises together from the head to the toes. You start with all the sitting exercises, then the standing exercises and finish with the strengthening and stretching exercises on the floor.

It is very important that you should have read every chapter in order to understand what you are doing to your body and why. There may be certain exercises which you need to do more often than others, for example the shoulder squeezes if you suffer from round shoulders or the tummy muscle exercises. Try and make these a part of your daily life and sprinkle them among your other activities. Put in *at least* one hour a week (preferably three one-hour sessions) to give attention to the whole body. Remember the body is a WHOLE. When you strengthen one part it is going to throw out the rest of the body, so you need to go through *everything*, even the exercises you don't like. You will probably not like them because they are hard for you, and they are most likely to be the ones you really need!

I have arranged the exercises in three columns. The first column is my basic class. The centre column is for people with bad backs and very weak tummies, etc., such as post-natal mums. The right-hand column puts in the harder exercises for you to progress to. Build up on the number of times you do each exercise, to increase your strength and stretch.

Use the basic class of exercise, then follow instructions in the centre or right column according to your needs. Do each exercise with your full attention and listen to your body each time. Don't worry if there are days when you seem unable to do anything right or when you find yourself stiffer than the last time you did the same exercise. The body has good days and bad days, so go all out on the good days and gently on the bad days. Remember that the bad days are usually the days when you least feel like exercising and sometimes the days when you most need it. There are no aerobic exercises included in this section, so it is up to you to run up the stairs, put on music you enjoy and jump or dance to it, run for the bus or for pleasure, play tennis or squash or do anything else that gets you comfortably out of breath AT LEAST once a day!

Don't expect miracles over night but above all DON'T GIVE UP. Your body is your life, so make it your priority. Staying healthy is more important than going to the shops or getting that report out. You are no good to yourself, your job or your family if you are only working at half your capacity, so don't let *anything* distract you or get in the way of *your time*.

EXERCISE CHART

BASIC CLASS	GENTLE CLASS	HARDER CLASS
Ex.	Ex.	Ex.
1 Pelvic tilts to correct sitting (page 15)		
2 Shoulder movements (pages 18, 27)		
3 First neck position – with hands (page 19)	3 without hands	3 with tilt and rounding forwards
4 Side neck release (page 24)	4 without hands	
5 Neck strengthener (pages 18, 22)		
6 Diagonal neck release (page 24)	6 without hands	
7 Arms up, push back (follow shoulder circles) (page 30)		
8 Arms up, push up (follow with shoulder circles) whole arm circles (follow with shoulder circles) (page 31)		
9 Shoulder squeeze (hands clasped behind) (page 29)		
10 'Chicken' exercise (page 31)		
11 Back of arm tightener (page 32)		
12 Arm rotation (page 32)		
13 Side bends (follow with shoulder circles) (page 69)	13 arms down	
14 Waist twists (page 70)		
15 Diagonal bends (follow with shoulder circles) (page 70)	15 don't do with a bad back	
16 Sitting leg kicks (pelvic tilt) (page 78)	16 sitting right back on stool	16 sitting on edge of stool
17 Ankle exercises (in and out) (page 111)		

BASIC CLASS	GENTLE CLASS	HARDER CLASS
Ex.	Ex.	Ex.
18 Buttocks squeeze (page 38)		
19 Buttocks squeeze, with legs raised (page 38)	19 buttocks squeeze, with feet on floor	19 go on as long as you can!
20 Pelvic tilt forwards – forwards bend to release (page 37)		
21 Foot exercises (toes and main arch) (page 121)		

Stand up by putting one foot in front of the other, body weight forwards and pushing off with your thighs, not heaving yourself up with your hands.

Now use the chair back, wall or table to stabilise you.

22 Strengthening the calves (feet together) (page 109)		
23 Calf stretch (page 105)		
		*24 thigh exercise 1 standing (page 86)
		*25 thigh exercise 2 standing (page 88)
26 Flat back release (bouncing on arms, with pelvic tilt) (page 89)	26 without arm bounce without arching back	
27 Standing quadriceps strengthener and stretch (page 80)	27 not if your knees are weak	
28 Inside thigh squeeze (page 90)		

Lying on the floor. Have cushion, belt or towel ready if necessary.

29 Pelvic tilt (with pelvic floor exercise) (pages 58, 73)		
30 Curl-ups (page 60)	30 don't lift more than shoulders off the ground	30 with arms folded or with hands behind head
31 Nose to toes (page 59)		

Roll head from side to side while supported on the floor after these exercises.

		32 Contractions (page 62)
33 Lying leg kicks (page 90)	33 use cushion under pelvis	
34 'The frog' (page 91)		
35 Legs apart in the air (page 91)	35 don't let legs drop forwards	35 pointed toes and flexed feet, legs apart and together

---

Bend knees to chest squeeze after these exercises.

36 Single leg lowering (page 65)	36 leave out if back or tummy weak	
		37 Double leg lowering and scissors (bend knees to chest, squeeze to release (page 67)
		38 Head to knee and elbow to knee (page 67)
39 Thigh exercise 1 lying down (bend knees to release) (page 83)		39 not if you did it standing up! (see 24)
		* as alternative to lying down

BASIC CLASS	GENTLE CLASS	HARDER CLASS
Ex.	Ex.	Ex.
40 Thigh exercise 2 lying down (bend knees to release (page 86)		
41 Bridge lift (pelvic tilt, hold and ripple down, try twice and then bend in knees to release) (page 39)	41 not if your back is too weak	41 with buttock squeeze and thigh squeeze, as many as you can then bend knees to release

Roll on to your tummy.

42 Leg lifts behind (pages 42, 45)	42 (use cushion) half bend single legs or straight single legs	42 set of four – take legs only halfway down between each lift

Turn head to the side, breathe to release between each exercise.

43 Leg lifts with legs apart (page 45)	43 single leg lifts, lifting leg up and outwards	43 set of 4 taking legs halfway down between each lift
44 Legs up and apart in the air *or*		
45 Legs up together, and down (page 45)		
		46 Legs apart, circles in and out (page 45)
47 Arm lifts (cushion away) with the top half (page 46)	47 single arm lifts	
48 Arm and leg lifted together (either with arms out in front or clasped behind back) (page 47)	48 lift right arm, left leg. left arm, right leg	
49 Ball position or rolling on back (page 44)		
50 Cat stretch (on hands and knees) (page 48)	50 don't arch, just contract and come back to flat back	
		51 Hinging (if you didn't do quadriceps standing, see 27) (page 81)
		52 Hinge release (if you didn't do quadriceps standing) (page 81)

Sit up.

53 Sitting with the soles of the feet together (page 95)	53 against wall until back is strong enough or with a cushion under your bottom	
54 Sitting with the legs apart (page 97)		54 pelvic roll to help pull back through
55 Hamstring stretch (with belt if necessary; stretched feet and flexed feet) (pages 77, 100)	55 lying on back with belt	
56 Curl-downs (page 63)		56 with hands behind head

Lie down on your back and have a rest!

57 The sideways pelvic tilt (page 48)
58 Bent knee rolling (page 49)

Ex. 53, 54 and 55 can be done before 29, with the curl-down leading into the pelvic tilt.